I0131723

This is a significant book. Combining first-hand experience as a "mental patient" with in-depth research, and sophisticated scholarship, Sharma offers a powerful challenge to the mental health establishment. Psychiatric diagnoses do not reflect reality, she argues, they create the idea that the distressed are mentally ill. Resulting from this diseasing of the distressed, is the erection of multiple barriers to recovery – interpersonal and institutional. In speaking sense to both the public and the professions – Sharma's analysis should stir broad dialogue and debate. This is the kind of scholarly activism that carries the seeds of social change.
–**Kenneth J Gergen**, *Senior Research Professor,*
Swarthmore College, USA

This book is a must-read challenge to the dominance of colonizing approaches to madness and distress. Drawing on Global South lived experience and knowledge, it offers fresh insights for challenging a maddening world.
–**Peter Beresford OBE**, *Visiting Professor, University*
of East Anglia, UK

Prateeksha Sharma gives us the hope that recovery from vulnerabilities and mental illness is possible without expensive psychiatric dogmatism. She makes it possible for the "patient" to reflect on the pain underneath the surface and how she/he can recover from the enduring struggles. I wish her the very best so that unadulterated joy can be ascertained with the thoughts of her book.
–**Anita Ghai**, *Professor, School of Human Studies,*
Ambedkar University, Delhi

With the lyricism and timing of a musician turned interdisciplinary researcher, Sharma's emancipatory scholarship draws us into deeper understandings of psychiatrisation and recovery. This book marks an important moment in the evolution of mad studies.
–**Bren LeFrançois**, *University Research Professor at*
Memorial University, Newfoundland, Canada

Language is not innocent! Sharma gives an impressive and thought-provoking account on recovery from psychosis, challenging the languages of the psy's. Reading this book and applying its ideas and concepts gives hope for a more socially just and inclusive society!
–**Ottar Ness**, *Professor of Counseling, Norwegian*
University of Science and Technology

Written against a backdrop of "diagnostic dominance", this book brings an emancipatory perspective to understanding recovery. Sharma sheds light on the ways people build a life around a diagnosis, how recovery often remains embroiled in psychiatric thinking, and the workings of power in governing people who won't comply.

–**China Mills**, *Senior Lecturer in Public Health, City, University of London*

BARRIERS TO RECOVERY FROM "PSYCHOSIS"

This book inaugurates the field of Mad Studies in the Indian subcontinent investigating the barriers to recovery from the perspective of "patients" and caregivers.

Offering a radical critique of the mental health system, it questions why the phenomenon of recovery from serious mental health issues is not more widespread. Drawing on narratives of "patients", evidence from lived experiences around the globe and literature on recovery in psychiatry, mental health legislations and policies, it establishes the hitherto silenced voice of the "patient" as having testimonial viability, via an emancipatory scholarship. It highlights the repeated marginalization of "patients" and the identity prejudice they experience in day-to-day situations as a form of epistemic violence. The book examines the barriers to recovery through an interdisciplinary investigation, scrutinizing relationships between individuals and institutions at interpersonal, intersocial and global levels.

The book will be of interest to researchers and scholars of psychiatry, psychology, anthropology, sociology, disability studies, Mad Studies, law and policy, cultural studies, mental health, medicine as well as general readers.

Prateeksha Sharma, psychotherapist-musicologist is the founder of Bright Side Family Counseling Center. Her counseling practice is informed both by her experiential perspectives and recovery research at the National Academy of Legal Studies and Research (Nalsar), Hyderabad. She works on interfaces between music, education, counseling, psychology and mental well-being among diverse demographics via advocacy, services, training and research.

BARRIERS TO RECOVERY FROM "PSYCHOSIS"

A Peer Investigation of Psychiatric Subjectivation

Prateeksha Sharma

Routledge
Taylor & Francis Group

LONDON AND NEW YORK

First published 2023
by Routledge
4 Park Square, Milton Park, Abingdon, Oxon OX14 4RN

and by Routledge
605 Third Avenue, New York, NY 10158

Routledge is an imprint of the Taylor & Francis Group, an informa business

© 2023 Prateeksha Sharma

The right of Prateeksha Sharma to be identified as author of this work has been asserted in accordance with sections 77 and 78 of the Copyright, Designs and Patents Act 1988.

All rights reserved. No part of this book may be reprinted or reproduced or utilised in any form or by any electronic, mechanical, or other means, now known or hereafter invented, including photocopying and recording, or in any information storage or retrieval system, without permission in writing from the publishers.

Trademark notice: Product or corporate names may be trademarks or registered trademarks, and are used only for identification and explanation without intent to infringe.

British Library Cataloguing-in-Publication Data
A catalogue record for this book is available from the British Library

Library of Congress Cataloging-in-Publication Data
A catalog record has been requested for this book

ISBN: 978-1-032-15832-7 (hbk)
ISBN: 978-1-032-16490-8 (pbk)
ISBN: 978-1-003-24880-4 (ebk)

DOI: 10.4324/9781003248804

Typeset in Sabon
by codeMantra

For my parents Subodh and Narender
who have always reminded that a life worth living
is lived for others and
peers, hoping my struggles will bolster yours

Only birth can conquer death – the birth, not of the old thing again, but of something new. Within the soul, within the body social, there must be – if we are to experience long survival – a continuous "recurrence of birth" (palingenesia) to nullify the unremitting recurrences of death. For it is by the means of our own victories, if we are not regenerated, that the work of Nemesis is wrought: doom breaks from the shell of our very virtue. Peace then is a snare; war is a snare; change is a snare; permanence a snare.

Joseph Campbell, 2008:11–12

From Joseph Campbell's *The Hero with a Thousand Faces* Copyright © Joseph Campbell Foundation (jcf.org) 2008. Used with permission

CONTENTS

Preface   xi
Foreword   xiii
Acknowledgements   xvii

PART I
Theoretical and methodological scaffolding   1

1   Recovery from "psychosis": realities and representations   3

2   Who speaks for whom and why it matters   29

3   Among peers, where one is home   56

PART II
Maps of recovery   71

4   "Benign" arm of psychiatry and birth of the
    psychiatric subject   73

5   From subject to agent *or* what it takes to recover   127

6   Making the transient permanent – how law impedes
    recovery   145

7   Decolonizing recognition   179

Appendix A: Demographic profiles of peers in this book   193
Appendix B: Flowcharts   195
Appendix C: From "treatment" towards disability   197

CONTENTS

Appendix D: The homeopathic mental
health establishment   201
References   206
Index   225

PREFACE

The story of this book has roots in my own life; the book started several years ago in my encounters with what is called "psychosis" by the psy-professions. To comprehend *barriers to recovery*, I had to myself take the path of *recovery from "psychosis"*, a slippery slope for anyone. Thereafter the effort became one of consolidating recovery: slipping again and again until a point was reached where I could avert *"psychosis"* by holding my spine straight and not letting life overwhelm me. The chronological order of writing this book pales into insignificance as pieces of my autobiographical journey punctuate the narrative of the book.

I cannot imagine the responses this book may evoke. But if I may, I hope to make this writing an invitation for dialogue. No doubt I have written many a word, or idea, or brought earlier ideas in newer formations but they would best be taken as a call to reconsider, reimagine, reconstruct. It has really taken me three decades to write this book. In that claim, there lies a surrender, no flourish; it is that long drawn a writing. Yes, experiencing the mental health labyrinth has taken time. Without it this work, and the different stages of gaining capacity for its synthesis, was difficult. But for those intervening stages this book would not have crystallized thus.

The terrain has been hazardous and unnerving for most parts. But there has been help, faith and encouragement. I have walked alone, invisible, but not entirely forsaken. In the year this book appears I am the load bearer of a half century of experience. If ever there were to be an audit of many un-accountable years may they be considered an investment of my youth, flesh and blood towards this book.

I stand in the role of the witness today – in time, of time. The past is over, yet shows up in stories of peers innumerably. The present is where I sow these seeds, with a hope that not just I but scores will change the course of their lives, even though when the brooding self surfaces,

> *"At times, in dark moments I wonder,*
> *Is it me who writes at all?*
> *Did I really sing in that concert hall?*

Did I dare walk the road without the milestone
Can I leave a footprint for another, a peer
Lost or losing, distant or near
Sister or brother who may with my dark or light
(whichever side they interact) effulgence
Interact, take a leaf, a spark, a blade of hope, a seed of inspiration"

When the songs still (Prateeksha Sharma,
unpublished poetry: 2014)

As the spring arrives and the moment belongs to birdsongs and multitudinous colours, there is a great sense of peace. I hail my peers, and others to whom "mental illness" matters to remind themselves what I say or write is what *we are all* capable of. I am nothing if not you/them. And if I can, so can you/they.

Prateeksha Sharma
Goa and Faridabad, February 2022

FOREWORD

The label of mental illness in law generally and in Indian law particularly has been associated with incompetence and dangerousness. This presumption created by lawmakers and reinforced by medical professionals has largely had an unchallenged existence. The challenge is non-existent because the primary stakeholder – the alleged "person with mental illness" or in legalese – the "person of unsound mind" – has been disqualified from speaking about self. Consequently others, that is medical and legal professionals, family and friends or even random strangers speak about them but their own voice is not even absently present. As the law is actively engaged in silencing the voice of the primary stakeholder, there is an all-pervasive silence on the lived reality of the person diagnosed with mental illness in law. It is this silence which Prateeksha Sharma breaks with her evidence-based, reasoned exposition on recovery. In doing so, Sharma has displaced the mental patient to introduce us to the human with all her fears and dreams; strengths and vulnerabilities; rebellions and oppressions. She has thereby shown that the story of the mental patient is not a story of illness and treatment. It is rather a tale of oppression and freedom; oppression perpetuated due to the uneasy concert between law, psychiatry, family and society.

This book is speaking about recovery as a real possibility for persons diagnosed with mental illness. It also finds that the diagnosis with its lifelong prognosis of having to live with the condition is the highest barrier to recovery. This central argument of the book caused me to ask: does law or even mental health law allow for recovery? The law I find envisages remission or lucid intervals but it does not provide for the fact of recovery. It seems to operate on the belief that once a "mental patient always a mental patient". Some illustrations demonstrating this fact may be useful. Thus, section 12 of the Indian Contract Act 1872 allows a person to contract during a lucid interval but not when of unsound mind. If a person is generally of unsound mind, then the burden of establishing that the contract was executed during a lucid interval is on the person defending the contract, and if the person is generally of sound mind, then the fact that the contract was entered into when the person's mind was not of sound mind lies on the party challenging the contract.

When it comes to institutionalization in psychiatric institutions, the law is again not speaking of recovery; it is only talking grounds and procedures by which a person could come in or go out. Institutionalization happens when a person needs institutional care and treatment and discharge is ordered when the person can be out in the world without any peril to self or others. Like the entry, the exit is also not an effort to make the inmate fit for life; it is only about deciding whether the person is fit to be discharged. This fitness is only assessed in terms of the individual and his or her psychological condition, or at best an exit into a less restrictive environment but the need to plan for the resumption of a full life is not envisaged. Following on Prateeksha Sharma's work, it is pertinent to ask: whether the absence of planning is due to negligence and callousness or because makers of both policy and law see no exit from patient-hood.

The deleterious effects of a diagnosis of mental illness can be further seen when the impact of non-disclosure on the right to marry and obtain employment is seen. Non-disclosure of a history of mental illness is seen as fraudulent in both employment and matrimonial law. One possible explanation could be that this diagnosis is seen to render a person dysfunctional; hence, any effort at trying to live an ordinary life is hindered by this legal expectation of disclosure. The irony is that if persons do not disclose, they are seen as fraudulent; and if they do employment is denied or marriage annulled.

The demand for truth in law is made oblivious of the stigma accompanying a diagnosis of mental illness. It is stigma rather than dishonesty which makes disclosure difficult. When non-disclosure is categorized as fraudulent, then the suffocation a closeted life gives rise to is waived away.[1] Persons diagnosed as mentally ill are mechanically viewed as baleful presences; Prateeksha Sharma in humanizing these struggles has asked some hard questions from psychiatry, law and society.

II

It is always easier to stop a harm which even the doer acknowledges as harmful. However, the paternalism which is extended to the psychiatric patient by both law and psychiatry is not seen as harmful but benevolent. Both legal and the medical initiatives are claimed to be beneficial for the patient and the person. Sharma's point in the book is that the patient subsumes the person. And it is this engulfing of the person in the persona of the patient she is questioning with the discourse and practice of recovery.

---

1 Karyakarte, K. "The Big Reveal or Looking for a Closet of My Own" paper presented in seminar course on Pluralizing Inclusion: Equality and Non Discrimination in a Globalizing World (NALSAR, October 2013).

Disability rights are as much asserted for adults as children. Child rights had to shake off the shackles of "the best interests of the child" and construct the concept of "evolving capacity of the child" to allow children to have a greater say in their own lives. The methodology of narrative inquiry that Prateeksha has employed in her work shows that there is a story; but for that story to be told empathetic listeners are needed. Such empathy is only felt in accepting and affectionate environments, not sceptical and suspicious ones. Sharma's work is asking how can infantilizing treatments produce responsible adults?

This infantilization is found in both medicine and law. The Mental Health Care Act in innumerable places allows the psychiatric patients being overridden by the psychiatrist (something which does not happen in physical health care) and yet the same statute requires ambulance services to psychiatrically ill persons on an equal basis with physically ill patients. This legal permission to overrule the patient encourages a non-listening relationship between doctor and patient. In the doctor-patient relationship, the balance of power is in favour of the doctor and the law instead of levelling the playing field further tilts the balance in favour of the doctor. The deference to medical judgement is not just provided for in the legislation; it also raises its head in adjudication.[2]

Thus, in Anamika Chawla's case, the Supreme Court did not even censure psychiatrists who ordered the compulsory commitment of the respondent on verbatim medical certificates without having physically examining the "alleged mentally ill person". And this result ensued even when the court quashed the reception order because they found the respondent to be of sound mind.[3] The judgement of Justice Muralidhar in *Ravinder* vs *NCT of Delhi*[4] is a rare case of the Court requiring mental health professionals to act in accordance with the law.

The legal resistance to giving up its *parens patriae* and colonial outlook is in full display in the recent judgement of the Madras High Court.[5] The Court was petitioned by the relative of a person with intellectual disability to appoint a guardian for his person and property. The Court notes that the new Mental Health Care Act 2017 does not allow for appointment of a guardian but instead of asking why such a change has occurred; it just concludes that by not enacting the guardianship provisions the legislature has created a gap and then swiftly fills the gap by relying upon clause 17 of the letters patent issued by the Crown to set up the High Court of Judicature at Madras. Persons with intellectual and psychosocial disabilities according to the Court must necessarily have a guardian even if to make such appoint-

2 See Dhanda, A. (2018). A Disability Studies Reading of Law for Persons with Disabilities in India. In Ghai, A. (ed.) *Disability in South Asia Knowledge and Experience*. Sage Publications.
3 Anamika Chawla vs Metropolitan Magistrate and Others MANU/SC/1186/1997.
4 MANU/DE/1548/2018.
5 C Raghuraman OP No 731 of 2021 decided on 27th January 2022.

ment the Court has to rely upon a nearly 200 years old legal instrument. The fact that such instrument has been prevailed over by both international and national law makes little difference to the Court.

A similar indifference Sharma finds when she examines the relationship between the UN Convention on the Rights of Persons with Disabilities (CRPD) and the Mental Health Care Act of 2017. She notes how the CRPD has been undermined by the Mental Health Legislation, which has done no more than create governance structures. Even if the law were to recognize agency, that agency is only conditionally provided. Both the law and the psy-establishment function as major barriers to recovery. Complete freedom or *purna swaraj* she holds requires each individual to struggle for their own vision of the world in recognition of the fact that "personal recoveries are triggered by micro environments".

III

This book can and will be read in several ways. Since it asks some very hard questions from law, psychiatry and society, it could be read to learn, or it could be read to refute and invalidate. Prateeksha Sharma is reporting her own experience and the experience of her peers in interaction with family and the medical establishment. These experiential reports can be accorded the respect they deserve because powerful establishments rarely get to hear what they are doing wrong. Or they could be dismissed as the opinion of a fringe minority. The numbers it could be pointed out are too small for these views to be taken seriously.

Psychiatry has for long claimed scientific status for itself. One of the characteristics of science is to scrutinize every evidence questioning its claims of truth. The suppression of the counter-view does not make the dominant view correct; it only makes it more powerful. In engaging with its critics every system gives itself an opportunity to undertake course correction. An efficacious remedy should not need coercion; rather, its efficaciousness should get people who need it to seek it. The author contends that by ousting competition, quelling dissent and mongering fear, the psy-establishment may have established suzerainty but should such sovereignty built on the enslavement of psy-patients through lifelong drug regimens be allowed to continue its enterprise unquestioned? Or should it be challenged? In answering this question in the affirmative, Prateeksha Sharma in this book has elaborated on the barriers to recovery and ways of striving for recovery and realizing it, a compelling argument which merits active engagement by all.

Amita Dhanda
Hyderabad, 25th February 2022

ACKNOWLEDGEMENTS

For the bouquet of ideas this book brings together my musical imagination may be held culpable. But I dare not stake claim for the work entirely for it has received many a support, door opened, invitation extended, critique and affirmation at different times, often beyond my imagination.

The reason this book got written is for the space opened up by Amita Dhanda at Nalsar University, with whom a chance encounter at the Medico Friend Circle meeting in Pune in 2015 created an opportunity to visit the university, and more doors that had been sealed on me for years suddenly opened. Yet the actual writing was shaped within my domestic walls, as my aging dogs breathed their last, one by one each year of this study. They were my immediate family – Raga, Nikki, Dash and Ginger who left from 2017 onwards. The loss would have been unbearable but for the new generation which grew up supporting this writing reach its desired end.

While the door was opened by one, it was another who ensured I did not run out of it the entire span. Without Ramakant Agnihotri, perhaps among the few in the world I have *never* hesitated to call, my ideas would never have reached fruition. His unconditional accessibility and unflinching support proved to me that everyone deserves a patient ear and just one gentle soul allaying their fears, biding them onwards. With a trusted mentor every David can take on a Goliath. For listening with wisdom honed over a lifetime I fall short of words to express my gratitude, not just to the person but equally the academic who facilitated my recognition of language, its significance beyond what I knew and for helping me through scores of methodological, ethical, linguistic, relational and philosophical dilemmas.

To the peers whose narratives appear in this book, so intimately part of the work that their voices and faces appear in front frequently, I am deeply indebted. Although to ensure their anonymity I cannot thank by name but because of that I am no less grateful. Many thanks to Rashna Imhasly-Gandhy for your presence, support, faith, and indicating ideational trajectories unthinkable once, especially in transpersonal psychology, analytical psychology and archetypal behaviour. It can be difficult for someone who has been at home for decades to do such work. Therefore, people who came in and helped from unimaginable quarters make me more humble as though it was a larger plan that I simply had to play my part in by staying long enough. Archana Parashar (didi) and Bhuvaneshwari Raman your early contributions have been invaluable. And to friends whom I turned towards at different times for different reasons, I am extremely thankful. In a scenario where all my interactions were on phone, for my solitary soul chipping away at unfamiliar ideas, your presence has been life affirming: Nalini Goyal, Chandramati, Monica Gupta, Subhash Chandra Malik (Bhashiji) for the earliest thumbs ups to my writing, and Anjali Capila for encouraging and feeling proud; it was so valuable. Jasna Russo you continue being the sole peer and sounding board for years. Your commitment to the global peer community is truly inspiring. And to peers in the Mad Studies group, believe it or not, when you all cheered me upon hearing the news of my doctoral degree I was deeply touched and immediately knew that there would be some who are ready to read whatever I had unearthed. Your voices to say the least have given me tremendous fortitude in going through all unlit, unnerving patches.

The role played by music is exceptional and my guru Smt. Madhuri Dandage has been a fount of encouragement, affirmation, accommodation, love and variety – diverting my mind with numerous *ragas* and *bandishes* depending upon my capacity for learning. Not to forget my students of music (and their parents) who learned for long or short durations, and remained my direct contact with the outside world during my years of introversion. My domestic space is a little oasis dotted with doggy barks, birdcalls, fish swimming, children singing, my own *riyaaz* (musical practice) and forays into backyard farming. In a reciprocal exchange I brought these disparate elements together and they created an ambience germinal for this book.

I am indebted to Dr. J.P. Kar for homeopathic support and Prinketu for supporting my spinal issues, for without resolving them it was not possible to work on the computer. Many thanks also to the Routledge editorial team: Lubna Irfan and Shloka Chauhan for your patience and support throughout.

I am once again grateful to my parents for shouldering the major burden of my domestic, intellectual and artistic activity. But for the spiritual, critical and musical sensibilities you raised us with this writing was unthinkable. My siblings have been there time and again to affirm how our core is as a family and what we are capable of surmounting when together. But also additional thanks to my brother Vikram – for the numerous books bought or sent via a diverse array of arrangements – including your friends travelling from the US. Perhaps it may be a moment of relief for you those efforts were not made in vain. And to my sister Sandeshika – for myriad forms of support from intellectual to gut and health issues, exercise to canine challenges – being there stoically, no matter the odds. And, yet again it is the dachshunds – Rhythm and Flow – the embodiment of furious activity in little bodies, whose doggy snores make me smile as I put this book to rest. And to the one who has taken a big hit for this work – Andre, I send a smile and a wink, hoping life will give us time to make up for it. Thank you for your fortitude regardless our circumstances.

I

THEORETICAL AND METHODOLOGICAL SCAFFOLDING

> I now believe that the biographical journeys of researchers
> greatly influence their values, their research questions, and
> the knowledge they construct. The knowledge they construct
> mirrors their life experiences and their values.
>
> James A. Banks (1998:4)

Is there an actual "mental illness" which afflicts people the way of another (somatic) disease? Can it be identified by tests or measures or does identification depend solely upon the person making the diagnosis? Do certain individuals or groups have greater tendency to "contract" "mental illness" while others don't? If one becomes "ill" is there no way to heal or recover? Who stands to gain if people remain "ill"? Do diagnostic labels help or cause more harm?

These uncomfortable questions are not raised in a world where someone's "mental illness" is accepted as incontrovertible proof by rhetorical tautology. Do epistemic and identity privileges not make some groups powerful over others, giving them unquestionable rights to create explanatory frameworks for the latter's behavior(s)? Is this not what colonial powers did in an erstwhile era?

The biographical aspects of this writing are the foundational structures of this section, and it informs all three chapters. An experience of understanding "mental illness" can bring vastly different outcomes in its comprehension and representation. This undercurrent is made explicit via the writing ahead.

This section flags these, among other dilemmas, in an investigation of "psychosis". Who is credible enough to interpret narratives of "mental illness"? Far from normative assumptions about "others" researchers' personal biographies impact research choices in emancipatory research and

DOI: 10.4324/9781003248804-1

such a framework is established in this section. The reader is invited to co-construct a methodological trail to evaluate whether the structure succeeds in shedding light on vast segments of humanity who suffer representational marginality due to widespread epistemic injustice. This book questions the social consensus about "patients" while establishing the nature of emancipatory struggles.

1

RECOVERY FROM "PSYCHOSIS"

Realities and representations

Although I shall be painting a somewhat depressing picture of language being increasingly caught up in domination and oppression, this will I hope be offset by my faith in the capacity of human beings to change what human beings have created. ... The more practical objective of this book is therefore to make a contribution to the general raising of consciousness of exploitative social relations, through focusing upon language.

Fairclough (1989:4)

ME: "You won't recover ... (do) you believe that?"
VINDHYA:[1] "Yes ma'am, I will not recover."
ME: "Because you have three diseases therefore you'll not recover, is that what (it is)?"

This dialogue between me and Vindhya has occurred in similar hues ever since we got acquainted. I wrote an article[2] advocating for recovery from mental health issues to be made a consideration of treatment goals. My email address at the end of the article led to several emails in response, her's among them. Over time we have become *friends* albeit in the interpersonal space created on the phone. We met once when I was visiting Hyderabad and she lived in the twin city of Secunderabad.[3] Our friendship has witnessed many a change in our respective lives since; though our recovery-oriented dialogues and her insistence on "patienthood" remain somewhat stable.

---

1 All names are changed to conceal contributors' identities, whether peer or parent. Author when appearing in dialogues is depicted as "me".
2 http://www.thehindu.com/todays-paper/tp-features/tp-openpage/complete-recovery-is-an-option-in-mental-illness-care-strategies/article6626080.ece.
3 This is not where she lives regularly but was there for a brief period.

DOI: 10.4324/9781003248804-2   3

VINDHYA: "Yes ma'am, for lupus doctor is telling … 'I myself don't know whether it will work out without the tablet, so you have to continue the tablets till your life … end of the life'."
ME: "Yes?"
VINDHYA: "So I am taking the tablets for lupus."

We are not discussing lupus but "schizophrenia" and the medications she has taken since the diagnosis, during her teenage.[4] Lupus and other gastrointestinal issues are the key side-effects she has developed over time. This book, however, is dedicated to investigating *recovery from "psychosis"*: an underlying condition of schizophrenia. While my inquiry is not confined to Vindhya, the dialogue above is the typical conversation we have had since 2014.

My writing begins from the *misrecognition* of distress as "psychosis" and consequences of the reification that follow. Does it help those recognized, and then, towards what end? Does recognition lead to resolution of distress or does it trigger something else instead, making people into lifelong "patients"? This examination is not done in neutrality, with a theoretical, scholarly curiosity, but with an emancipatory perspective – derived from having been the subject of such (mis)recognition.

Vindhya and I, we are peers. The latter has overcome barriers which prevent a majority from recovery and the former hopes for something identical. In her email she inquired whether she could recover. I responded in the affirmative; a response informed by experience. My courage came from "the idea of 'recovery', which has recently come to prominence in policy internationally. Its appeal has lain in its promise that survivors would not be written off as forever useless" (Beresford, 2016:27). I had little idea back then, when we started talking, what could hold someone back in the mental health system; this inquiry was not even on the horizon. I was simply keen to offer my testimony to anyone who would heed to the idea, or me, and willing to explore options which may offer succour and healing.

People recover from serious "mental illness", including "schizophrenia" and "bipolar disorder", though not frequently. A diagnosis of "psychosis", no matter how damning or bewildering, is *not* a final verdict on a person's life. Yet the preceding dialogue exhibits how Vindhya, like a vast number of people given a psychiatric diagnosis, take their label as finality and build a life around the belief of its permanence. I myself did so for 18 years. Vindhya's self-conception as "patient" runs like a red thread, an exemplar of a typical "patient", throughout this book. Having taken a stable "patient" identity, she does not question her anchorage in a worldview which no longer helps, or regardless what evidence, knowledge, peer

---

4 At the time of this dialogue we were both in our mid-forties.

support, co-morbidities come her way. An "expert's" recognition of her suffering serves to reconfigure distress as "illness". Recognition from others is thus essential to the development of a sense of self; in this case a "patient" self. To be denied recognition – or to be "misrecognized" – is to suffer both a distortion of one's relation to one's self and an injury to one's identity (Fraser, 2000:109). Whether or not this recognition amounts to misrecognition is what we examine ahead.

Having a long past of "bipolar disorder" I understand both "psychosis" and recovery intimately. There are few domains in which I have spent more time than I have in what is commonly called "mental illness". At 20 years, I was diagnosed "bipolar in disorder" but uncharacteristically also exited psychiatry nearly two decades later, something which eventually helped me recover. While personal recovery[5] is a starting point defining the politics of my scholarship, I utilize my illness narrative as marker to reveal my *positionality*. In addition to mine the reader will encounter two other kinds of narratives in this book: references to third-person narratives already in the public domain, and narratives gathered especially for this study.

From where I begin: a question of positionality

My past of being in the "patient's" role, its social and political context (Holmes, 2020:1) constitutes my positionality and establishes the origins of this study and its agenda while my opinions, values, beliefs and social background (Manohar et al., 2017:2) influence the process, shaping each methodological and analytical decision. Lived experience imparts me an emancipatory sensibility to investigate this issue in a specific manner.

By yardsticks of academia people like me are "minority scholars", or "insider-outsider" in research. I am an "insider" of being labeled "manic depressed" or "bipolar in disorder". I see myself as "peer" to those already recovered, or who continue to look for alternatives or who have accepted the "patient" status. Our experiences unite us though I try gaining comprehension of "psychosis" and recovery just as others pursue other trades and professions. Being currently outside of the frame of "psychosis" and equally my peers' lives I become an "outsider"; researcher, not "researched". From a plethora of choices[6] of similar work in mental health this effort is most appropriately defined as emancipatory or *survivor* research. Citing Lucy Costa, Sweeney (2016:36) suggests that just like Mad Studies,[7] in survivor

---

5 I have written about it from the year 2011 onward, citations ahead.
6 Sweeney (2016:36) uses the phrase survivor research from among synonymous phrases like survivor-controlled research, survivor-led research, service user-controlled research, and service user-led research. I prefer to use no survivor based terminology but refer to it to indicate my location in research or who my natural allies are.
7 A detailed exposition follows ahead.

research too no single person, or school, or group owns or defines its borders. How different ideas are developing is also shaped by geography and experiences of the mental health system among other factors, and this may reflect as diverse epistemological and ontological positions.

The attitude of revealing one's position is central to such efforts as mine and researchers attest to its credibility (Pasquini and Olaniyan, 2004, Mellor et al., 2014, Stiedenroth, 2014), power, knowledge construction and representation (Merriam et al., 2001:406). Positionality acknowledges and recognizes that researchers are part of the social world they are researching and this world has already been interpreted by existing social actors (Holmes, 2020:3). In the present case the world I attempt re-interpreting belongs to the individual labeled "psychotic", "psychosis" itself a psychiatric representation. In psychiatric terms deep emotional turmoil and distress are classified "psychosis", such suffering long reconstituted "illness". But just because it has been called so does not *make it an illness*. Our unequal social world damages a majority of people and ecology due to inherent injustice, greed, power imbalances and imposition of hegemonic epistemic regimes on people with lesser power to create counter epistemologies. In recognition of such structural injustice and to create an alternative representation, directly articulating the experiences of "patients" mine is but a small effort.

Following Savin-Baden and Major (2013:71–73) my positionality is tripartite: *survivor research* in research parlance, having proximal understanding of the mental health system as it operates in India. Second, in relation to the contributors of this book a *peer*. The opening lines offer a glimpse of my peer role, yet this perception is equivocal for experience teaches me how prejudice and stigma may work against the former "patient". Third, being a peer I represent others as an equal, not specialist, barring my (researcher) role and (academic) location.

My context: social representation of peers and unravelling their (our) governance.

Representation, research and praxis in mental health

Researchers in mental health span a wide spectrum – from psychiatric professionals to other psy-professionals: psychologists, clinical psychologists, psychotherapists, psychiatric social workers, human scientists – sociologists, anthropologists, legal scholars to cultural, language and disability scholars. This book is not rooted in any one traditional[8] discipline as a majority of recent researches (Bindhu Lakshmi, 2006, Borg, 2007, Addlakha, 2008,

---

8 The predominant tradition of research in mental health is normative or positivist research by psychiatry and interpretive research by scholars in other human sciences.

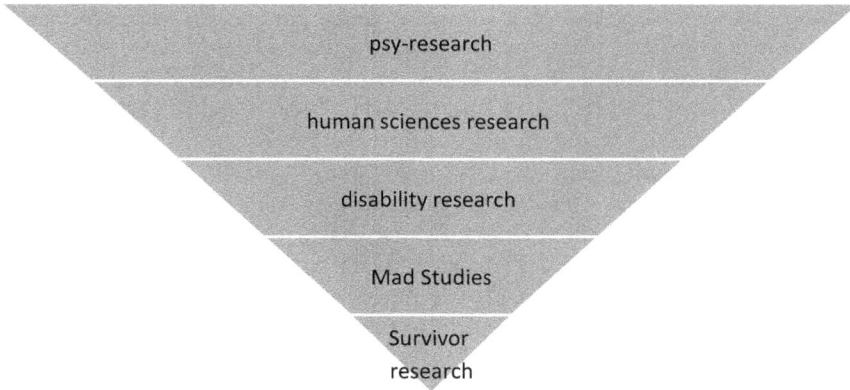

Figure 1.1 A representation of the diversity of fields associated with mental health research

Ranganathan, 2011, Law, 2014, Larsen, 2016, Mathias, 2016, Llewellyn-Beardsley et al., 2019, Yarris and Ponting, 2019, Sommer et al., 2021). These researchers are scholars working as clinicians, psychologists, social workers and sociologists – anthropologists among others. While they speak of the "mentally ill" with empathy, their goals are either normative or interpretive: to represent subjective realities of "patients". Some problematize the biomedical stance of "mental illness" as "unhelpful". Yet the ontological assumption remains there is a state of *being* "mentally ill" or some medical condition which is not easy to comprehend except for a biomedical explanation.

A majority of these scholars have not experienced any "mental health" issues that evoke diagnostic labels; their work constitutes third-person psychology. Those who have such experiences construe distress differently, rejecting the biomedical view of our suffering (Diamond, 2012, Voronka, 2015, Johnston, 2019, Russo, 2019). We are "insiders" or *minority scholars*. Making this positionality explicit helps me situate my book in the larger discipline of mental health research done by people who critically assess their experiences of the system, via an emerging field called Mad Studies and sets the tone of my politics, opposed to taking an "illness" view of suffering (see Figure 1.1).

Self-representation – "Mad", "survivor" or "emancipatory"

The struggle to choose a suitable representation for myself is a long one for I seem to have a ready pool of neologisms encapsulating my kind of experiences: "Mad", "psychiatric survivor", "ex-patient", "consumer/survivor/ex-user"[9] or more. Some differences emanate from ontological assumptions, and some from our linguistic preferences. I am neither at ease with any of these words nor intend to limit my struggles against oppression to mental health. I favour the word "emancipatory" for myself; not even "survivor" for that too has a prefix of psychiatry: "psychiatric survivor"! I have no intention of tying my identity with an oppressor! For me emancipation connotes radical politics, decoloniality and recognition of oppression beyond identity politics or essentialism. "Emancipatory – (x)" is my preferred home. The "x" may be any suffix: peer, academic, activist, therapist or another. Emancipation is the goal, rooted in liberatory ideas, quest for knowledge, moral capacity and constant struggle to identify oppression.

When I settled to work on this book, I did not feel like an "ex-patient" or "survivor" but someone who emancipated herself from diagnostic dominance. What else is emancipation if not recognition of oppression, a struggle to wrest free? As long as we having a past/present of deep distress do not represent our oppressions and injustice the world will only believe expert-led views of our realities attributing ideas and constructs which resonate with us but little. It is primarily through representations in academia, society, media, law and policy landscapes or elsewhere, we will reclaim our personhood and rights, speak for the silent or silenced, and start sowing seeds of change among professionals, peers, caregivers and other stakeholders. Possibly then we may forge some alternative to hegemonic and enfeebling psychiatric discourse.

There is no such thing as a value-free investigation of social reality; transparency and attentiveness to the investigator's own standpoint are critical for the whole research process, starting from its design (Russo and Wallcraft, 2011: 215). Before delineating the contours of my inquiry, including its design, I would like to clarify the linguistic choices about representing myself, and how I settled for it in the presence of alternatives.

My research falls into the category of emancipatory peer research, starting from visualizing research contributors as equals. While there is an element of representing others, it is equally a representation of something personally experienced for decades. My research, understandably, is unlike a majority of researches in mental health: it is not value neutral. It has a definite set of values, goals and agendas. "There are extensive accounts written from the perspective of mental health professionals about

---

9 The word "user" is used interchangeably with "consumer" in mental health literatures to denote someone utilizing psychiatric services, as though people have a range of services to choose from and whatever they choose is really a matter of choice!

patients/consumers/survivors … And yet, there are relatively few sto-ries about suffering of service users from their own perspectives" (Lee, 2013:105).

In as much as we are peers, I cannot deny or ignore that a degree of in-equality between the researcher and the researched may be characteristic of any kind of research (Bindhu Lakshmi, 2006:3). While aware of this I have tried inculcating awareness, reflexivity, acknowledging how my past and present are often sources of a diverse set of emotions, such as curiosity, interest, confusion, unsettling, doubt, misgiving, mistrust and possibly eva-siveness both in me and among peers. I repeatedly endeavour not to alienate peers from this work by ongoing interactions wherever feasible.

My position mirrors closely what people given psychiatric diagnoses in many parts of the world are attempting "through grassroots democratic action into what was initially referred to as 'mental patients' liberation", and later as "c/s/x" (consumer/survivor/ex-patient) movement (in North America) and the "psychiatric survivor" or "service user" movement (in the United Kingdom)" (LeFrancois et al., 2013:6). None of this phraseol-ogy emanates from India, where the ground reality is somewhat different. Whatever opposition to psychiatry is present in India it is confined to few activists and/or scholars, whose work remains geographically restricted and/or within academic domains, beyond the reach of the "average"[10] "patient". When I was a "patient", I never encountered anything inform-ing me about psychiatry's violence, violations or hollow promises. There is massive ignorance about psychiatry's oppressive role in society and peo-ple often visualize it as a benign saviour, unless they have faced forcible "treatments" themselves.

It may surprise someone that psychiatric "patienthood" is associated with disability, for the average person does not consider "patienthood" dis-abling. We often see disability in "the other", the one visibly so. But by accepting oneself to be "mentally ill" one inadvertently becomes disabled: alienated from the world, unable to have access to a majority of things others freely do – living without medication, following routines determined by work and professions, earning livelihoods, forging relationships, being socially active.

I myself did not understand this for at least 25 years, ignorant how invisi-ble barriers held me from "being normal"! I could neither accept how I was disabled by a label nor acknowledge any aspect of my disability or knew its nature. While I deal with disabling aspects of "psychosis" further on for the moment my goal is to situate this book within the ambit of disability studies, as a foundational, though peripheral, pillar.

---

10 I often refer to the typical psychiatric patient as the "average" patient and count myself among them, not to be seen in a pejorative sense.

From disability studies to "Mad"[11] studies

Russo and Beresford (2014:153) note over the last generation disability has been transformed by the emergence of new discourses challenging longstanding dominant medicalized individual discourse, due to impetus from disabled people themselves. They have been based on experiential knowledge – people knowing about disability directly through experiencing impairment and being on the receiving end of disabling attitudes and barriers. Unlike the non-disabled perspectives ... the Disability Studies Approach centralizes the voice of persons with disabilities, while challenging the primacy accorded to the allegedly objective knowledge possessed by professionals of the human mind and body (Dhanda, 2018:385).

Undoubtedly, disability studies is a valuable starting point but "mental illness" and its location within the framework of disability studies is not an altogether straightforward case. We need to distinguish the nature of disability for investigating people disabled by psychiatric "patienthood". Disability Studies believes in the ontological reality of "mental illness", a view those opposed to psychiatry reject. Consequently, we offer a critical view of psychiatry's knowledge and an experiential view of our suffering – both due to the inherent distress and the experience of the psychiatric system. This effort is currently crystallizing in the form of Mad Studies. An ontological rejection of the "biomedical" basis of mental health issues is a point of departure between Mad Studies and disability studies.

Mad Studies is an emerging academic field of study comprised of activists and scholars who share similar critiques of psychiatry (Brewer, 2018:14). In recent years, disability studies publications have increasingly included perspectives on psychiatric disability. Any disability studies journal routinely publishes articles on madness along with work on physical and sensory disabilities; this was not the case even 15 years ago (ibid:12). It builds on a compelling tradition of critical activism and scholarship, which open up a wealth of opportunity for 21st-century struggle against psychiatry in its many forms (Menzies et al., 2013). Mad Studies offers a real prospect of effective opposition to the marginalization and oppression of experiencing madness and distress, which is strongly philosophically and intellectually grounded (Beresford, 2022:1). Spandler and Poursanidou (2019:3) affirm that critically examining the dominance of the psy-disciplines and discourses is certainly a key component of the Mad Studies project, without which there is a risk of collusion with top-down professionalized understandings of madness and distress.

---

11 The word "Mad" in "Mad" studies is always represented in uppercase to indicate it is not really a project of "madness" or belief in biological psychiatry but a project of being "Mad" in the sense of being angry or reclaiming oneself from oppression.

Within the broader scope of disability studies, though this writing aligns with Mad Studies, more precisely my perspective mirrors most closely those who identify as and do *survivor* research. Both Mad Studies and survivor research are emerging fields ... whose goals and boundaries are being continuously shaped (Sweeney, 2016). The word "survivor" is a euphemism not my preferred self-representation. Yet I still choose to identify with this group of activists and academics hoping that goals of resistance will supersede our linguistic choices and divergences. Survivor research can be considered the systematic investigation of issues of importance to survivors, from our perspectives and based on our experiences, leading to the generation of new, transferable, knowledge (Sweeney, 2016:37).

My preference for emancipatory research over any other morphological variant also lies in my belief that "mental illness" is not a real category of "illness", except being a discursive, representational reality. When people are forced (or obliged) to take psychiatric "treatments", akin to "becoming subjects of psychiatry" (see Chapter 2), they are disabled *per force*, not because they were born with or "contracted" a disabling "illness".[12] An imposition of the biomedical view catalyses transition of distress to "disease". To situate such inquiry within disability studies does little justice to people who are at the receiving end of a system which does not address issues of distress except for a treatment recommendation. Before someone enters into psychiatric "patienthood", they may seem simply "odd" or non-conforming, not necessarily "disabled". While disability studies focuses on building a radical critique of barriers to disabled people's inclusion in society, Mad Studies examines society's structural aspects which lead people to having breakdowns, the manner they become psychiatric subjects or remain so.

This is not to suggest that mental suffering does not disable people, for chronic suffering certainly makes people dependent, feeble and unable to cope with life alienated from the world around. But the promise with which psychiatry enters our lives does not match up to reality; it does not relieve suffering. Instead "treatments" worsen health condition over time, or produce comorbidities at the very least. In a nutshell, psychiatric "treatments" far from healing push one towards disability! My insistence on choosing Mad Studies over disability studies is not to be construed as making disability studies meaningless for people with mental health issues. I must clarify that

[w]hen we choose not to name our relationships to disability in our scholarship, we limit opportunities to serve as role models and to

---

12 This may be equally true for any disability. The emancipatory view of disability acknowledges that disability is not a medical or personal problem, as much as it is a social and political project wherein people are disabled less due to what they are born with and more by prevalent social, attitudinal and normative barriers. For further reading see Oliver (1990, 1992), Shakespeare (2018).

build community because others simply do not know why we have come to the field or how we imagine it.

(Brewer, 2018:27)

Notwithstanding hesitation of embracing a disability identity, my work banks in significant ways on emancipatory voices of scores of disability activists and academics, and I cannot but concede how I myself have been disabled over the past three decades.

Richard Ingram (2008) coined the phrase "Mad Studies":[13] perspectives based on a transformative revaluation of the category of "Madness". This was an extension of the disability studies perspective offered in the belief that the reality of people who are forced to take psychiatric medication cannot be adequately represented in the generalized concept of disability. The idea behind giving the name Mad Studies to certain perspectives is intended to set a minimum threshold for academic investigations to be considered as offering radical critiques and alternatives to psychiatric, psychotherapeutic and psychological perspectives, whose pathologization of madness as "mental illness" entails wide-ranging negative social and political consequences (Ingram, 2008:1). Ever since the publication of *Mad Matters* (LeFrancois et al., 2013) from Canada where this newly emergent area took off, it has had a watershed effect internationally (Beresford and Russo, 2016:1). Kalathil and Crepaz-Keay (in Russo and Beresford, 2015:153) propose that "the work of mad-identified scholars and activists can be seen as balancing the overwhelming majority of material written about those who are labelled mad by those who do the labelling and those who study them". These perspectives have been historically and systemically undermined if not entirely dismissed from consideration within dominant psy-professions and disciplines that maintain a hegemonic position of authority within policy, practice, knowledge, law and service for those who use mental health and disability services (Joseph, 2019:2).

For Fabris (in Menzies et al., 2013:11), "'Mad' is an historical rather than a descriptive or essential category, proposed for political action and discussion". In many ways, I resonate with the idea but still hesitate in embracing the "Mad" label, lest it be construed as essentializing or an

---

13 He proposed this nomenclature in a presentation made at an undergraduate Disability Studies Symposium at the Syracuse University in 2008. He remarks: "particularities of surviving – living on – as psychiatrized people are not adequately reflected by a generalized concept of "disability". Just as Deaf studies has claimed spaces at least partially autonomous from those of disability studies, so Mad studies requires its own partially autonomous spaces. The purpose of these other spaces is not to fracture disability studies into multiple, discrete disciplines. Instead, the power knowledge assemblages of Deaf studies and Mad studies need to develop on the basis of their specificities, in addition to exploring communalities under the over-arching heading of disability studies" (Ingram, 2008:1).

identity assertion. I have said elsewhere (Sharma, 2022:342) "Mad" as idea or response to an oppression has only a symbolic presence in our (Indian) society, and then not in a truly radical, emancipatory or visionary manner, but an identity category that a few like to uphold. Therefore, I embrace the resistance, the critical perspective that Mad Studies offers, but steer clear of identity politics including survivor research, just as Mad Studies has been conceptualized – a democratic resistance offering flexibility to choose one's tools. From my Mad Studies-based approach, I straightaway move to language and its complexity in the field of mental health.

My politics begins with positionality and sends trajectories in diverse directions. Foremost among them is the role of language, central to this writing. I attempt to communicate equally to the stakeholder as the student, to the professional as much as "patient". Consequently, I draw attention towards themes around language throughout.

> To language the sciences entrust the duty of depicting or mirroring the results of their inquiry. It is language, then, that must bear objective truth ... And if it is language that carries truth across cultures and into the future, one might reasonably conclude that species survival is dependent upon the functioning of language.
>
> (Gergen, 1997:31)

The recognition it is language which dominates and via language a whole epistemological-ontological complex governs people occupies a central role in this book. While I may be ill-fitted to offer a critique of language, my focus lies on outcomes it produces in people's governance. It is a question of our survival in spite of distress produced by life's injustices, which makes this inquiry pertinent. I have grown up with a fondness for verbal and artistic communication, which may explain this urge to examine the roots of social intercourse. My idea is to problematize language itself, so the quantum of distress is not amplified in the name of serving us, veiled in words misrepresenting our lived realities.

Language concerns

It was the role of language and its discovery via social constructionist scholarship (Gergen, 1997; Fee, 2000) which made me awaken to a "discourse of deficit" in representation of people in distress.

> [W]e are unlikely to question the existence of the reality to which such terms seem to refer; and because the prevailing ontology of mental life remains generally unchallenged, we seldom inquire into the utility or desirability of such terms in daily life.
>
> (Gergen, 1997:147)

13

This realization proved like a paradigm shift "akin to Gestalt shifts in perception" (Kuhn, 1962:111) becoming the starting point of change in my personal narrative. Therefore, language occupies a unique position in this book beginning with its role in producing recognition, and being the medium of representation.

Representing "madness"

The word "madness" is mostly ascribed to a state of someone's experience and produces recognition of a specific kind in the mind of the listener. But what if this representation does not mean anything except producing *that* recognition?

> From the pragmatic perspective it is of paramount importance, then, to inquire into the effects of the prevailing vocabularies of the mind on human relationships. Given our goals for human betterment, do these vocabularies facilitate or obstruct? And ... what kinds of social patterns does the existing vocabulary of psychological deficit facilitate (or prevent).
>
> (Gergen, 1997:147)

While Gergen questions the utility of certain vocabularies, their effects on people who become identified with these vocabularies are less than salubrious. The role of such identifiers is confined to labelling "such people" and managing them.

It should come as little surprise that some would like to reclaim the term "madness" from diagnostic reductionism, whereas others believe psychiatry itself is "a regime of ruling" (Smith, in Burstow, 2013:79), which gives names (labels) to others, or in fact "words cannot be seen as innocent" (ibid:81). Burstow also believes that part of the conceptualization work facing us (researchers and activists) involves creating critiques that problematize the discourse underpinning this regime. I have used language in this spirit: by *not* accepting psychiatric language unquestioningly, only tactically – putting it within scare quotes ("..."), to express my disagreement with such representations. Let us be warned by Burstow (2013) about the perils of using psychiatric terminology, for it reifies biomedical categories as "truths", they are not. Foregrounding this perspective as foundational to my approach, I clarify my use of certain words and phrases:
Diagnostic labels – "Mental illness", "psychosis", "schizophrenia" and "bipolar disorder" represent "illness" categories based on psychiatric ontology. They may not be maps of an existing truth or reality. By using these words, I neither accept their "illness" claim nor ontological basis. I utilize diagnostic words to produce a verbal and symbolic recognition and unambiguity since all stakeholders understand them. It simplifies the message.

I even use these words interchangeably without signifying difference. These categories do not represent a measurable, material reality "treatable" by pharmaceutical cures.

"Patient" – "Patient" is indicated within commas, for it denotes the belief of being patient than *having a treatable illness*. By this, I do not intend to dismiss someone's suffering as imaginary. Suffering is real, heartfelt and experiential. But *calling* it an illness does not make it one. The *becoming of a patient* is also something that I delve in later (see Chapter 2).

Psy-professionals – Nikolas Rose coined this phrase to represent psychiatrists, clinical psychologists, psychiatric social workers and psychiatric nurses as people who derive their knowledge and professional claim due to their belief in biological psychiatry. Diamond (2013:76) notes it is not sufficient to simply refer to psychiatry, given that in contemporary times, many related professions are greatly influenced by the psychiatric paradigm and in many ways complicit in maintaining psychiatric hegemony.

Peer research – I assign myself the role of a *peer*, and this study amounts to peer engagement or knowledge, performed among people who understand "psychosis". In psychiatric services, whenever "peer" is employed, it denotes a current patient. The preferred use among scholars like me is "survivor" and such research as "survivor-controlled" or "survivor-led". As I said earlier, I hesitate to identify as "survivor" and explain ahead how my use of the word "peer" is a deliberation at disrupting how research is produced.

What makes me write this book

Two reasons may explain the reason behind this effort. First, psychiatric morbidity diminishes the quality of life of those suffering and their caregivers. It has deleterious outcomes for society if people of a healthy and potentially productive age group become dependent on others instead of being well enough to contribute their best to their social worlds. Yet this is not part of a neoliberal agenda identifying people as "productive bodies" – grist in the societal mill, who simply produce goods and services serving financial interests of global corporations. Mine is an effort at unravelling the process of subduing and governing "discomfort-producing", non-compliant people. Such individuals threaten the status quo-oriented social fabric which demands unchallenged submission from citizens, punishing anyone who falls out of line from their assigned or expected role(s).

My goal is unsettling the marginalization of vast numbers of people and their reduction to passive consumers of psychiatric goods and services, dismissing their suffering as subjective, non-viable babble. Instead of seeing people as "mentally ill" and believing they deserve a medical "treatment", there may be other ways to conceptualize emotional turmoil. Distress-producing conditions can be resolved in empowering ways, rather than pushing people into actual disability. Herein lays the first rationale for studying these potentially disabling conditions from the "patient" perspective. Principally, I scrutinize aspects of the (subjectivation) process and identify pathways to diminish the suffering psychiatric "patienthood" spawns.

My second argument comes from social representations, a subfield of social psychology. Moscovici (in Breakwell, 1993) suggests that social groups generate representations which serve group purposes. Representations serve different types of group interests, and he describes three: diffusion, propagation and propaganda. Diagnostic labels are social representations by a dominant group of another (oppressed) group which lacks the ability or means to counter it. The powerful group achieves its dominance due to its ability to establish its knowledge as a source of power,[14] discursively constructed within members of the group. Thereafter, this knowledge is diffused to the rest of society and propagated further becoming part of common sense social discourse. Inasmuch as dominant groups can represent subordinate groups, the latter can also represent themselves. As an emancipatory researcher, I offer peer narratives, analysed via a linguistic lens, as counter to psychiatric conceptualization of us as "mentally ill" subjects. Mine is an alternative social representation[15] of the same phenomenon. The overarching sensibility "is based upon my assumption that social science, as an area of inquiry like therapy, has understanding and improving the human condition as its goal" (McNamee, 1989:95).

Setting the agenda

This work is a response to the state of "treatments" whereby people who seek ways out of suffering not only sink further but also end up becoming disabled due to the "help" they receive. This is where I lean into Disability Studies (DS) for the rights of people with disabilities enters the frame. But not only "patients" whole families plunge into despair, for a majority in India relies upon families for all kind of help, as elaborated ahead (Chapters 4 and 5).

Diverse groups, in their convergent and divergent struggles, engage in emancipatory struggles against what we recognize our oppression. This recognition takes long to crystallize for the well-oiled mental health machinery befuddles everyone until the realization dawns that "treatments" are unhelpful, not bringing transformative outcomes. If one recalls my opening dialogue with Vindhya, three decades of "treatment" and progressive disability have not dimmed her faith in the medical model. "[W]hat if psychiatry itself mobilizes a colonial relation, alienating people from their

---

14 I discuss this in Chapter 2 as epistemic privilege.
15 Davar (2013) also points towards the significance of representation and political participation of the mentally ill.

own understandings of distress and violently interpellating them into a 'fixed' identity as 'mentally ill'" (Mills, 2014:136)?

Once such realization occurs more often than not those who struggle against the "treatment" regimens are stymied due to lack of resources, especially the kind it takes to create an epistemic response to the hegemon. The distinctiveness of what we have to say continues to be re-framed, neutralized and even erased in ever more sophisticated ways (Russo, 2016:60). "[W]e as survivors, with support from our allies, must advance our knowledges, ideas and theories to bring about a very different future for all" (Beresford, 2016:28). Even though we may exit the mental health system as individuals, sometimes a personal struggle[16] is dwarfed in the face of suffering of millions not permitting conscience to rest easy. Hitting the nail on the head, this book has a "future forming" (Gergen, 2014:2) intent. Lest mistaken, I should clarify the intended future is *not* based on continued, unchallenged epistemic privilege of the normative "expert". Instead, it is one where every truth, however deemed by "experts", is worthy of recognition and generating a befitting social response. A future that emancipatory researchers envision belongs to egalitarianism not hegemony, radical democracy not deafening disciplinary rhetoric, epistemic and cultural plurality not homogeneity and no overarching models with a global broad sweep but cultural, local and individual answers to daily micro-aggressions against peoples.

My position emerges from a rejection of diagnostic neutrality and its biochemical basis whereby some chemical whose lack is causing the distress, if identified correctly and provided to the optimum dosage, would henceforth bring relief. Though many constituencies counter this perspective especially those within psychiatry having critical psychiatry perspectives (Healy, 2006; Summerfield, 2012, 2013; Moncrieff, 2013; etc.), my origin lies in experienced reality. My ontological view: "mental illness" is a socially constructed truth, which morphs into an "illness" serving (certain) group interests.

The writing ahead unfolds from here and presents the bases of these claims or whether they stand the test of credibility. *What lies ahead may not please for it is not even a goal.* My goal is to examine social power meant to signal an epistemic authority, manifested through language use in day-to-day professional practices. I explicate how diagnostic evaluation and subsequent labelling cause harm to individuals they claim to "serve".

Distress as "mental illness" – who is being served?

Human distress when classified "illness" by psychiatry has immense power to shape public opinion, where after this classification acquires a status of

---

16 This is a key reason I could not leave the field of mental health behind even though I could have created a career in music.

truth, becoming ontological reality. Gergen (2001:12) pointing towards the constructed nature of "truth" says while we may all agree that there is something unusual about an individual's behaviour, why should we suppose that the community of clinicians and psychiatrists are correct in calling it "mental illness", and that DSM[17] categories are maps of this world.

> [D]esignating suffering as a medical problem diminishes the ability of an individual or group to describe and act on it politically. The increasing prevalence of mental disorder, and correlatedly psychiatric concepts, means that these concerns have perhaps never been more urgent for those of us who are interested in political agency and citizenship.
>
> Degerman (2020:1)

> The point is that the prestige of the scientist ... can be used to lend power to its possessor. He then may be able to achieve social goals that he could not otherwise attain.
>
> Szasz (1974/2010:26)

Instead of confirming this deficit-based conceptualization of people's distress and accepting diagnostic labels, I explore a *holistic*, rather than an *atomistic* approach to mental disturbances. This approach is likely to place such disturbances out in the world of everyday life, rather than as a dysfunction solely within an individual (Shotter, 2016:1). I do not suggest that people's suffering is insignificant or they cannot be deeply impaired by it. Instead, in support of my ontological position, I advance the idea that genesis of "mental illness" can be probed in people's subjective life situations, instead of biology or behaviours implicated by psychiatric epistemology.

Going by this ontology, how can one see what is called "mental illness" and how should it be recovered from? The actual question is whose knowledge about recovery counts? Should we examine recovery from the point of view of psychiatrists, caregivers or "patients"? Epistemology is after all a question of *who can be a knower*. For me, it becomes an issue of *who can decide about recovery*, or how this knowledge can be acquired. I explain later (Chapter 2) why the overarching framework of this book comes from social construction. In a constructionist frame, all research constructs the world in its terms. The major question is not of objectivity, but of utility. For what purpose is the research to be used (Gergen, 2009:71)?

---

17 DSM: Diagnostic and Statistical Manual of the American Psychiatric Association, seen as the Bible of psychiatry and utilized by psychiatric professions all across the world to define diagnostic categories.

In the context of qualitative research, Parker (2005:20) notes that representation may also be seen as making a position statement, especially how those one researches are represented. In the context of this research, he refers to two kinds of representations: (a) referring to another and (b) self-reference. He proposes the first to find alternative ways of referring to what we used to call "subjects", and to accord them agency in the research as "research participants"; my preferred phrase being *research contributors*. The second aspect is in terms of self-reference the researcher uses, with one key marker of this self-reference in qualitative research being to write in the first person – to take responsibility for what one did and to position oneself by saying that "I did this". It is due to this spirit of agency and responsibility the first-person voice is audible throughout the book.

Personal context

My entry into "mental illness" occurred in 1992, an unconscious stumble into a bewildering, stigma-ridden reality. I was in the final year of an undergraduate degree when a prolonged melancholia plunged me into "manic depression" (the term "bipolar disorder" appeared later). Back then, there were no avenues, unlike today, to understand the meaning of a diagnosis. It was as though a bolt from the blue struck me and my family. The setback derailed me for months as neuroleptics numbed my mind so deeply I could not graduate with my batch mates, but a year later. That pronouncement took a massive toll in the initial years. From then onwards till November 2010, I predominantly believed myself to be a "patient", albeit in a private invisible domain. While pervasive stigma silenced me about a part of my life, a general unawareness about mental health issues further necessitated the silence; for who wants to give lengthy explanations to another whose world seems far removed from such dismal realities?

Two near simultaneous occurrences 18 years later, in 2010, brought a shift in my self-perception as a "mentally ill" subject. One was the discovery of social construction and its critique of "mental illness", via dispersal of a dominant discourse and another, a chance encounter with a homeopathic physician. On the one hand, my moods and their upheavals as I quit psychiatric medication were managed by homeopathy; the shift in my philosophical worldview was mediated by social construction. Neither was I a "patient" in a short time nor felt victimized, helpless, overwhelmed and isolated carrying the burden of a shameful, stigmatizing identity.

Yet, strangely enough what I thought was left behind in 2010 suddenly caught up with me towards the end of 2015. I was suddenly engulfed by the familiar eddies of "psychosis" that had vanished for long. It was in some part due to the anxiety of getting into doctoral research coupled with other relocation-related stressors I had been unmindful of. By then, my family[18] had a lot of experience of handling such crises; it was mitigated in a few weeks.

Gaining comprehension about recovery

In three decades from 1992, I have spent significant parts of my adult life around issues of mental health, in changing roles – medically, socially, emotionally, professionally, ontologically and philosophically. Over time, my interest has morphed from looking at the meaning of diagnostic categories to looking for further evidence how these categories are determined at all. I have been tracing contours of recovery and its politics, forging a capability to question the rhetorical, philosophical and epistemic basis of "mental illness". This shift has been incremental – at times arithmetic, at times geometric. I no longer hear narratives of "illness" in an ideological vacuum but also sniff the sociological contexts which harbour their germinal conditions. It is precisely these contexts which also define the contours of someone's recovery: the principal proposition of this book.

There was a time recovery from serious "mental illness" was unheard of. In the decades starting the 1970s, this phenomenon began to appear around the world. As it began gaining attention, it became significant, albeit with little consensus, among different constituencies. Knowing its complexities and uncertainties, I was keen to look for its societal acceptance, among related issues. For one thing in all my years of "patienthood", I did not know someone could recover from "bipolar disorder". There was no community to fall back on and periodic visits to any psychiatrist (who would be) hard pressed for time and was an unlikely door to new knowledge except consolidation of their confirmation bias.

My journey of comprehending recovery began when I quit psychiatric medication (in 2010) yet its epistemic basis remained embroiled in psychiatric ontology. I mark this as the first phase of my understanding, when I was trying to capture personal recovery via research. Writing personal accounts helped me rebuild myself after psychiatry and make sense of an experience that had been frightening and unspeakable for a very long time (Russo, 2016:59). Reading my autoethnographic writing (Sharma, 2011, 2014, 2015), one encounters a "patient" talking about "bipolar", time and again, as though trying to establish recovery as personal (even though emancipatory) triumph. There was no idea of questioning ontology, though social construction had planted a seed of doubt.

---

18 I make this point about my family because inadvertently someone experiencing "psychosis" is unable to deal with the immediate crisis. They need support by others who understand, and are willing to step-in till the one distressed is safely out of the emergency. When this happened I was living with four dogs in a city on the outskirts of South Goa.

Matters of identity are hard to displace often taking a form where identification with classificatory paradigms is axiomatic. It was later, in the second part of my endeavours to do recovery research, when I moved to a social context. When I got interested in the phenomenon on a bigger canvas, beyond the personal, this change in perception began to occur. A personal story may even be an egoistic claim, but if/when we are able to see the patterns of the personal in a wider context: identify oppression as a social reality the emancipatory vision begins to integrate.

Even though I have researched into many aspects of my recovery, working with others' narratives imparts the analytical process distance, objectivity and scope for newer synthesis. Interestingly, psychiatry itself has been course correcting for the last several decades, partially in response to new values, dilemmas, questions, ethics and evidence and partially due to the appearance of recovered people offering testimonial evidence. Meanwhile my writing opened rehabilitation avenues and options for leaving the abject world of the lonely "mentally ill" by connecting with others, reach out to kindred souls. But not without paying the price of years spent in terrifying and disabling anxieties, in the iron prison of a perpetually foggy mind, spinning endless calamity-ridden scenarios. The disability could have lasted forever yet strangely enough when I stopped psychiatric medication everything changed. There were severe withdrawal effects but also support from many quarters. Having known psychiatric disability intimately I cannot but marvel at anyone who manages to overcome it. It makes me curious to know its pathway in their story.

Nature of psychiatric disability

Disabilities are defined as an inability or limitation to perform tasks expected of an individual within a social environment (Thara and Rajkumar, 1993:33). What is it about "mental illnesses" which makes them disabling, especially when people are initially able enough to seek help for their suffering, recognizing their need to heal, get respite? The disabilities of persons with schizophrenia can be very severe, encompassing the entire gamut of an individual's personal, social and occupational functioning (ibid.). Whether disability can be located within the biology (mind & body) of the individual or their life history is of the essence.

When I look at experience in hindsight, memory of overwhelming anxiety flashes instantly, coupled with fog in the brain, generalized sense of loss, apathy and grief peeping out from those years. It was paralyzing fear not allowing taking up or sustaining a job which I tried variously, building a career in a sustained manner – which my association with music could have engendered, or work out a marital relationship in a stable fashion – which the joint family system does not foster for the "mentally ill" woman. There

21

was no semblance of "normalcy" in any domain. "Failure" stared without respite – for more than 20 years. To varying degrees, this experience is echoed by a majority.

> This story now seems symbolic of how disabled I felt taking psychiatric drugs. They never worked well for me. Partly this was because I was forced to have chlorpromazine against my will several times, which felt like a terrible assault. It led to blackouts, amnesia and a general uncomfortable feeling of being strangely divorced from the world around me. During another hospitalisation I was made to take haloperidol, which had the effect of sending muscles in my neck and face into spasms so that my head was twisted violently, my face made grotesque masks, while my teeth ground together as if they'd break. On other occasions the spasms extended to my back so that I was thrown to the floor as if by an invisible wrestler ... Nurses at first thought I was "acting out" and didn't believe this was the effect of the drug. I think this shows how little the people who administer drugs know about the effects they have.
>
> (Simpson, 2016:152)

For professionals, the nature of disability can be an objective evaluation of people's functioning in different domains of life/work. Seen from the perspective of "patients", it is the helplessness of one's situation and the effects of drugs, which are most disabling. Forcible drug "treatment" is itself a trauma, over and above the primary suffering that drives anyone towards psychiatry. Such "help" entrenches one's helplessness and powerlessness more so. Longitudinal studies have shown that the disability associated with schizophrenia improves over time, but the contribution of antipsychotic treatment to this is unclear (Tirthalli et al., 2008:2).

Straightforward as it may appear recovery is *not* a natural prognosis for a "psychosis" diagnoses. The preponderant idea is a life of a "patient" – playing the "sick role".[19] An acceptance of being "ill" after receiving a psychiatric diagnosis is a norm. It is noteworthy that becoming a "patient" is vital for what such *becoming* translates into. It has a bearing on life ahead for it opens up two options: (a) actually "being" or (b) "believing" oneself to be "mentally ill" (see Chapter 2). The questions of why it is important to the field of "mental health", what is to be recovered or how I situate this work are discussed later.

---

19 Used in medical sociology this phrase was first suggested by Talcott Parsons in 1951.

Encountering peers[20]

The first article I wrote (Sharma, 2011) itself opened new doors of connections by putting me in touch with others who had been given similar or other diagnoses. At a later date, I would be approaching these people as peers to invite into this study. Until then, I did not know a single other for years, with any "mental illness" diagnosis – an ignorance which caused me immense grief, implanting my self-stigma further and making loneliness ineradicable. Meeting and listening to peers seemed a relief and our voices resonated for once. We saw our reflections in one another and for a span of time the connections seemed welcoming and heartfelt.

But attempts of gathering narratives among peers made me encounter a different reality: not only was I seen as an exception due to recovery, my success was additionally attributed to being a musician. I was told[21] since I had accomplished something unheard of it was not because recovery is a universal possibility but because I had access to resources others did not. Nevertheless, those efforts put me in touch with scores of others across India, via social networks of Facebook, emails, personal meetings, with people and organizations, and invitations to speak in institutions of higher education. Not only peers writing also connected me with caregivers around India, as well as non-profits working in mental health, other researchers and diverse activists. At the time of planning this project, I thought I had a ready pool of people to fall back on, as potential contributors. Suffice to say my rehabilitation exercises of writing put me in a larger social context, and continues enlarging.

The preceding paragraphs briefly map the pathway of my diagnosis, its disabling aspects and reaching a stage where it slipped into the past due to rehabilitation. The initial research in recovery brought me to the next stage – from the individual to the social context of recovery and whether there were common strands across recovery and/or illness narratives.

What is "psychosis", and recovery?

The roots of the word "psychosis" lie in neurology and the word was coined by the Austrian physician Baron Ernst Von Feuchtersleben in the mid-19th century. The term seeks its origin from the Greek goddess of the soul or spirit, Psyche, whose name *psukhe* personified "the breath of life". The

20 I utilize "peer" in a different manner than psychiatry employs it, by referring to people who are current "patients". My usage suggests my attempt to equalize research and social relationships with people who are given "mental illness" diagnosis. Since we come from similar experiences my relationship is not merely a traditional researcher's, interested in gathering others' narratives one-sidedly, as I share further into the book.
21 A caregiver, also involved with a non-profit, told me so.

derivative term *psukhosis* referred to a state of animation. Daniel Tuke (in 1892) defined psychoses as mental affections, including states of consciousness, thoughts and ideas (Sommer, 2011:162–163).

While I don't believe what psychiatry classifies as "psychosis" is a "treatable" condition capable of being medically "cured"; my rejection still acknowledges that for many it is a truth having its basis in experience. It appears unexplainable due to lack of explanatory capacity of one having the experience. Therefore, I use psychiatric terminology, even though problematizing it throughout. For psychiatrists, "psychosis" is a certainty around which they build considerable theory, themselves unsure about it!

Given that psychotic disorders affect 1%–3% of the population and rank among the top 10 causes of disability worldwide (van Os and Kapur, 2009), predicting psychosis has become a priority in the international mental health field over the past two decades.(Benoit et al., 2019:20–21). This is so even while admitting that psychiatry has not yet discovered the natural boundaries of psychosis. Psychiatrists van Os and Tamminga (2010:xxi) as part of their attempt at deconstructing it propose that psychiatry can only observe its properties, and "the only way to achieve progress is to periodically reassess all the evidence in the hope of catching a glimpse of its natural pathology". Though psychiatrists are still not clear about it, millions are routinely diagnosed with "psychosis". When people are diagnosed and psychiatry lacks clarity how to "treat" it to produce healing, talking about recovery becomes even more controversial.

It is another matter that there is enough scholarship which questions the basis of psychiatric diagnosis (e.g., Scheff, 1999; Rogers and Pilgrim, 2005; Goetzche, 2015; Cohen, 2016). It challenges the necessity of classifying individual suffering by heaping stigmatizing labels on people, instead of helping them deal with it befittingly. The recovery I investigate comes from this attitude – to recover from the effect of going through the psychiatric system and labeled "mentally ill".

Recovery is not altogether an unproblematic or unquestioned idea in the wider realm of mental health, for there is a spectrum of opinions, views, studies, claims and dismissals of the notion of recovery (see Chapter 2). For now, the idea holds a minor, somewhat insignificant position in the mental health discourse prevalent in India, equally as much in popular imagination as in government policy. But this does not mean that recoveries cannot or do not happen – people recover from a diagnosis of "psychosis" in India by taking different paths. No doubt one does not hear much about these recoveries because it remains a stigmatized area and few want to talk about something painful or embarrassing they have already put behind them. As one of my research contributors (Jitendra) told me, "*after years of being well and fully functional, one does not feel like talking about it often, equally so in hindsight*".

24

"Mental illness": reality or representation?

In the entire duration of my personal experiences and then research, the stark reality that stands out is "mental illness" is widely, rather unambiguously understood in India, regardless what language represents it. I personally do not[22] accept the word "mad", "madness", "mental illness" or the idea that there is a chemical lack within a person, which can be accurately identified and "corrected" by suitable biomedical means. Unlike researchers who use phrases like "severe mental distress" (Borg, 2007), I problematize an "illness" based construction.

Language is not value neutral, and understanding its importance is central to an endeavour to understand the meaning of people's suffering and their representation. From the linguistic turn in the social sciences, and by understanding that experience is discursively constructed and construed, "mental illness" to me is a matter of representation embedded in a differential of social power. Further ahead, in Chapter 2, I will discuss this in detail. For now, I enter the field by saying that I view language as the chief fulcrum on which the (power) relationships between people rest. I concur with Fairclough that ideology is pervasively present in language. And therefore it ought to mean that the ideological nature of language should be one of the major themes of modern social science. Nobody who has an interest in modern society, and certainly nobody who has an interest in relationships of power in modern society, can afford to ignore language (Fairclough, 1989:3).

Not only a medium of representing others language is also the mode of self-representations, social positions and politics. I have already stated above the meanings of the words, as I use them, how I differentiate between how they are commonly utilized, where I derive my position from and whether/how they reflect the current work done by emancipatory researchers.

Organization of chapters

This book has two sections: theoretical and methodological. For a study re-creating the structural barebones, making explicit the manner it is conducted and its findings arrived at is justifiably expected. A reader may not be keen about the planning of this book and its research details. To such an individual, I recommend straightaway going to the second section, where narratives and the mental health law are analysed. After reading those if it piques your interest to engage with the theoretical ideas underpinning this writing, you are welcome back to section I.

---

22 This is not to say that I always held this position. For almost two decades of life, I believed in "psychosis"; like another believing myself to be "mentally ill".

My method is a dual analysis of (a) "patient" and caregivers narratives, and (b) extant provisions for recovery in law and policy of India. The reader may be reminded that while mental health concepts are laid down by psychiatry, their implementation is carried out via legal and policy decisions empowered to create institutional mechanisms. It appears reasonable to examine popular social, individual and medical perceptions and understandings about recovery, probe the changes required in legislations to create a scope for recoveries, and whether or how to harmonize the laws with the UN-CRPD.

One goal of this writing is to use social science research to provide an evidence base that may influence policy, legislation and the decisions courts make (Cashmore and Parkinson, 2014:239). This effort is best seen as creating recommendations for modifying procedures and making suitable changes in laws governing psychiatric practices.

The theoretical scaffolding of this book, in Chapter 2, extends the writing in this chapter and my experience of the mental health system. I start by analysing whether experience is a valid starting point for an emancipatory project. I deliberate upon how this conceptualization makes all the difference in the representations one makes. Thereafter, I attempt to understand the concept of recovery, seen from diverse positions of psychiatry and people with insider's experience. In the following segment, I investigate how or why psychiatric conceptions of "mental illness" become hegemonic and what mechanism(s) catalyse this dominance. Bringing these into the framework of philosophy, I work through the notion of epistemic injustice proposed by Miranda Fricker (2007) to visualize how this form of injustice marginalizes certain groups in society, privileging others. The overarching framework of this study comes from social construction and I explain its contours in the context of this work.

In Chapter 3, I narrate how the peer role changed the manner in which this research was conducted, as compared to other research in mental health. I write about negotiating challenges of gathering data and attempting an emancipatory sensibility (Oliver, 1992) aimed to disrupt the social relations of research production. Using the framework of critical discourse analysis to analyse narratives, my eye is on how power plays out socially through language, marginalizing certain people and establishing or reinforcing certain other hierarchies.

I have chosen qualitative research, a way of learning about social reality (Leavy, 2014:2), to examine micro-aspects of recovery. Such minute details can only be extracted by looking at individuals closely, paying heed to them, engaging, interacting and exchanging ideas at close quarters. Such questions cannot be asked via a fixed questionnaire or rigidly defined responses; individual lives being different and beyond the imagination of any researcher.

In the social and behavioral sciences, these approaches to research are often used to explore, describe, or explain social phenomenon;

unpack the meanings people ascribe to activities, situations, events, or artefacts; build a depth of understanding about some aspect of social life.

(ibid.)

Qualitative research is an umbrella term for a wide variety of approaches to and methods for the study of natural social life. The information or data collected and analysed is primarily non-quantitative in character, consisting of textual materials such as interview transcripts, field notes and documents (Saldana, 2011:3).

Understanding why recovery is not widespread necessitates a closer scrutiny of the culture withholding its proliferation. This goal can only be reached by examining what people do to recover and wherein the gaps lie. For these goals, a qualitative in-depth study of a few people's stories seems like a more appropriate form of gathering facts; people like us are not found easily or in large numbers anywhere. Qualitative design is more suitable for this work as they use representative sampling strategies to make inferences about a whole population while producing maximum theoretical understanding of a social process (Faugier and Sargeant, 1997:791).

From the narratives of 18 people,[23] the qualitative data of this book, I have identified a few themes to investigate more closely why people seek psychiatric help upon experiencing distress. Since my investigation is into *barriers to recovery*, I propose them as a bivariate. In Chapter 4, I examine the first set of variables identifying them as *micro*-barriers. They lie concealed in the micropolitics of mental health as it occurs within day-to-day domestic and other interpersonal spaces.

The second set of variables – the *macro*-barriers to recovery – lie within legal-policy landscapes. I scrutinize them in Chapter 6 wherein all instruments are analysed. In the Indian Mental Healthcare Act 2017 (MHCA), recovery is not mentioned as a goal of mental health legislation, yet the law is called "progressive", creating outcomes that do not necessarily further the interests of "patients". I write this chapter in continuation of my earlier narratives, setting them against the contours of contemporaneous legislations, to study how law and policy impede recovery. If recovery is not even a legislative objective does law only assist more people become "patients"?

The Convention of Rights for Persons with Disability (CRPD or Convention) is an international convention of the United Nations (UN), in whose passage and formulation people with disabilities have played a significant role. The Convention is considered as a set of laws which are legally binding on signatories: member nations of the UN. In this chapter, I comb through the MHCA to examine whether it upholds the CRPD in spirit. If it does

---

23 These are ten "patient" and eight caregivers' narratives.

not, how could law be changed, so it may harmonize with the CRPD since India ratified it? My position affords me the opportunity to see both legal provisions theoretically (in law and policy) and their daily functioning on the ground (in my own life when I needed them, and professionally in others). When law creates a host of options, are they actually present for people as options when they require mental health services?

By writing this chapter, I extend an opportunity for the legal and policy community to comprehend the picture beyond the dominant view of psychiatrists, who are most vociferous and at the forefront in the passage of this (retrograde) law. I represent our "patient" perspectives: for whom these laws are passed, services created. If people are unable to recover notwithstanding legal provisions, (forced to) remain "patients" by a milieu which does not create sufficient recovery options, then clearly mental health legislation fails its purpose. It cannot uphold their rights or values enshrined in the CRPD.

It is not as though the absence of enabling environments hinders recovery entirely. Chapter 5 documents narratives of recovered peers. In Chapter 4, their narratives had similar contours as everyone in a "patient's" role. In Chapter 5 their narratives turn towards healing and recovery; outcomes of their agency and extant medical pluralism. People recover in unexpected ways yet there are common strands running across narratives and the role of family gives new insights. This helps distinguish differences between families where recoveries occur and where they do not.

Does psychiatric recognition help the suffering individual? Who is served most by this classification, and does it lead to desired outcomes for those who sought ways out of their distress? Building on evidence from previous chapters, Chapter 7 advances the need to decolonize recognition. It both summarizes the barriers to recovery from "psychosis", and proposes a way forward building on epistemological decentring. What does it mean for "patients" and families and where do future trajectories lie? What about "Mad" and emancipatory perspectives? Apart from theoretical areas, there are other possibilities in disparate domains, which may follow from this writing. Some are discussed in the concluding chapter.

2

WHO SPEAKS FOR WHOM AND
WHY IT MATTERS

[T]he linguistic-conceptual ordering of the phenomena we
call "diseases" and of the interventions we call "treatments" –
is a human activity, governed by human interests.

Szasz (2007:xviii)

Does experience count?

Defining "experience" is vitally important to decide which voice can represent it. As someone who understands "patienthood", I cannot but fore-
ground the personal albeit clarifying what it refers to. If I were to say mine
was an experience of *being mentally ill* as opposed to *being a subject of
psychiatry*[1], these are markedly different views, leading to radically different understandings. This choice, of which experience is referred to, makes
a difference in representations of "experience" and births varying politics,
of those who testify for either.

There are caveats and caution recommended in seeking to study experience or believing it always amounts to knowledge. When experience is
taken as the origin of knowledge, the vision of the individual subject (the
person who had the experience or the historian who recounts it) becomes
the bedrock of evidence on which explanation is built (Scott, 1991:777).
In a mental health context, if I say I have experience of "mental illness",
I implicitly accept the basis of the claim: there is indeed a "mental illness",
an objective category, whose experience I allude to. A stance of accepting
"being mentally ill" reifies "mental illness", justifying Scott's (1991:777)
caution: taking as "self-evident the identities of those whose experience is

---

1 Foucault (1982) distinguishes the idea of the "subject" in two ways. The first is in the
  sense of "made subject to" as done by control or dependence. The second "made subjects" is tied to the idea of subjective identities, produced by being "tied" to a specific
  who or what they understand themselves to be, is "made" or produced by being "tied" to
  a specific identity through a "conscience or self-knowledge". I develop the latter of these
  ideas more fully in a following section of this chapter.

DOI: 10.4324/9781003248804-3   29

being documented and thus naturalize their difference". The experience of *being mentally ill* confirms psychiatry's biomedical view that there is an objective state of "mental illness", that exists before the treatment and it can be treated through invasive biomedical intervention (Pattadath, 2016:203).

Experience: "illness", or coloniality?

Simply put if one says the experience is of *being a subject of psychiatry*, it necessitates another conceptualization: by viewing it as a form of coloniality. "I invoke a historical perspective here" (Gergen, 2007:149) to distinguish colonialism from coloniality and interrogate how "our discourse for the self is ontologically secure" (ibid). Coloniality has become a crucial theoretical resource for scholars across a range of disciplines (De Lissovoy and Fregoso Bailon, 2019:83) and my goal is to turn towards the psychiatrist– "patient" relationship with this lens. The notion of coloniality of power emphasizes the distinction between colonialism (a concrete social formation) and coloniality (an encompassing political, cultural, epistemological and symbolic condition) (ibid.).

> Modern colonialism instituted enduring hierarchies of subjects and knowledges – the colonizer and the colonized, the Occidental and the Oriental, the civilized and the primitive, the scientific and the superstitious, the developed and the underdeveloped. The scholarship in different disciplines has made us all too aware that such dichotomies reduced complex differences and interactions to the binary (self/other) logic of colonial power.
>
> Gyan Prakash (1995:3)

While extraction-focused colonizers eyed colonies for their natural resources and economic opportunities, they simultaneously imposed their knowledge(s) and worldviews on the colonized. "History became the product of the West in its actions upon others" (Bhambra, 2014:116). In recent years, scholarship in different disciplines has vigorously traced the relationship between the formation of authoritative knowledge and the exercise of colonial power that denied other people knowledge and agency (Gyan Prakash, 1995:10). Foucault has referred to these epistemic assessments as hegemony-seeking versus subjugated knowledge (Alcoff, 2007:80).

There are three things to be distinguished here – while colonialism is a visible political structure, coloniality is the active reduction of people as governable entities. The latter remains tied to power and even in the absence of a colonial government such institutions and structures can prevail well after the emergence of the independent state. Gonzalez Casanova (1965) calls this internal colonialism.

The explanatory framework adopted by psychiatry to respond to people's emotional crises is akin to the colonizers, about which Jara and Pisani (2020:334) note "the Eurocentric colonialism of biomedicine and psychiatry becomes visible by imposing some forms of knowledge on others and exerting political control strategies in subaltern groups, such as the mentally ill, women and indigenous peoples, among others". Nandy (2009) and Porter (2015) help develop this reasoning further: an important buttress of colonizing forces within psychiatry is the assumption that psychiatric disorders are discoverable facts of nature that transcend questions of social interest (Porter, 2015:5–6). Regardless, a feasibility of such discovery by other means the underlying idea is that psychiatric "experts" have the power to speak about "patients" (now subjects) as though their mind-body is the "territory" of psychiatry, to be dealt with in accordance with the judgment of the former.

This reconfiguring of distress as diagnosis marks the start of the psychiatrist-"patient" relationship, based on the assumption that the former can ameliorate the condition of the latter which she hardly comprehends. The "patient" on her part wants to identify closer with the educated, social class psychiatry represents and willingly embraces the biomedical view of her suffering, further adopting its language representing her distress as a *superior way of knowing* herself. Kiossev (1995) wonders whether such cultural characteristics cannot be classified "self-colonizing", which import alien values and civilizational models by themselves and people lovingly colonize their own authenticity through these foreign models. In a similar fashion by taking distress away from its social context, and recognizing it as an authentic response to systemic oppression, through the biomedical framework, the "patient" pushes it away at a biological distance – alienating both herself from her oppressive truth and a (mis)recognition that it *lies within* not outside, in the social milieu.

Nandy (2009:2) notes that colonialism is a psychological state first of all and carries a certain cultural baggage. In the colonial culture, identification with the aggressor bound the rulers and the ruled in an unbreakable dyadic relationship. When India was a colony the (British) Raj saw Indians as crypto-barbarians who needed to further civilize themselves. It saw British rule as an agent of progress and as a mission. Many Indians in turn saw their salvation in becoming more like the British (Nandy, 2009:7). In this representation, if one were to substitute the word "psychiatry" instead of the "British" and "patient" instead of "Indians", the pattern becomes self-evident. Lugones (in Potter, 2015) also confirms that colonizing does not just involve classification of people into unequal kinds but also the process of active reduction of people, the dehumanization that fits them for the classification, the attempt to turn the colonized into less than human beings. What the consequences of this reduction are is explained by the ideas of epistemic privilege and epistemic injustice, further on.

Though lived experience is the first epistemic pillar of this study, the idea is not altogether unproblematic. Voronka (2016) and Pattadath (2016) warn of the flip side of making lived experience a claim to expertise, knowledge and representativeness of an entire spectrum of "mental illness". The vastness of experience spanning a whole range of oppression based on location, gender, race, disability and other variables need not be encapsulated in another (normative) essentializing category called "lived experience". The claim to representing a wide population based on a personal lived experience is complicated.

Yet, instead of seeing this as essentializing experience like Scott (1991), I draw attention to those previously marginalized by history and offer that this rewriting of history has produced a wealth of new evidence previously ignored about these "others", and often many of the things they have to say are unworthy of mention in conventional histories. Commenting on the value of efforts such as mine, she confirms that "these histories have provided evidence for a world of alternative values and practices whose existence gives the lie to hegemonic constructions of social worlds" (Scott, 1991:776). At the same time, she reminds us that the "visible is privileged", and seeing is the origin of knowing. Until something is visible, it cannot be known, and visibility is gained only by becoming transparent. Therefore, those who have "experience" need to speak for themselves and for the experiences they have/had.

A second argument is offered by Voronka (2016:189) who problematizes the manner in which people are selected to represent lived experiences of mental health, calling the process slow and uneven. She notes from her activism and representation of lived experience that organizations that seek

> participation remained rooted in conservative and paternalistic values. Psychiatric survivors and the more radically marginalized are usually not recruited; instead, those who called themselves "consumers" and those more or less appeased by the mental health services they had received were the first to be chosen to sit, speak, and represent on various boards, in consultations, and on panels.
>
> (Costa et al., 2012:90)

O'Donnell et al. (2019:1–2) also express frustration that people who share their stories remain disadvantaged, often unpaid, unequal partners while organizations, professionals and academics benefit through receiving funding and building a career path on the basis of user involvement.

Extending the argument whether experience can contribute towards an emancipatory theory building, lived experience in an unequal society too often lacks an awareness of the need to struggle against privilege (Lather, 1986:262). This nods towards Voronka about who gets to represent lived experience. It further raises the question whose experiential perspective can speak for a whole community of "patients", accommodating diversity and intersectional oppressions. Yet in what manner can one expect a better system of mental health services for the vast majority of people if it does not include representations of those who have been wronged, suppressed, mistreated, silenced, epistemically marginalized or who question/oppose the system? In such a varied scenario, the questions become – whose experience and what/if such experience can contribute towards social justice?

Mere speaking from lived experiences does not amount to an emancipatory struggle as representation may not have a goal beyond identity politics. Lived experience can diverge into diverse politics, emancipatory struggle only one among them. Keeping emancipation as a goal has both epistemic and methodological implications. On the epistemic side how we respond to "peers" and maintain their representation(s) as central to our academic ventures reflects both a relational stance and commitment to community. Experience is an ethical compass for engaging others as equals, while their unmediated testimonies are representations beyond labels they are summarized by.

I bring this emancipatory sensibility here. Since the goals of emancipatory knowledge and resistance are clear to researchers who speak from experience, our methods and approaches are decidedly different from those who speak from similar experience with support offered by social privileges or from making essentialist claims. My goal is to represent a phenomenon closely experienced bringing forth peers' testimonies without doubting or letting their representations be lost among a din of other voices.

Whose experience matters

There are diverse stakeholders of "lived experience" or "experts by experience" as family caregivers are extremely active in India, at the forefront of mental health advocacy, representation and activism. Along with mental health activists, who speak for greater access to psychiatric services, and a rights-driven model of mental health, a majority of biomedicine-oriented stakeholders press for greater psychiatric access. Many identify as "users", "consumers" and "experts by experience", being past or current patients. So, when I respond to the question: "which experience" I distinguish between two groups.

The first group "patients" believe they are "mentally ill", while the second, more critical (Mad Studies oriented) people, believe we had "experience of the psychiatric system" and somehow wrested free. Belief in "patienthood" reifies "mental illness", whereas a search for solutions makes us examine the distress produced by daily oppressions, an area which merits examination. Such critique points towards a new epistemology – decoding the politics of daily living and its mental health outcomes, setting one free from a self-sabotaging identity.

33

Reading large bodies of narratives, autobiographies, memoirs and research of and by people who have been "subjects" of the psychiatric system, one notices a rich countercurrent flowing in the world of the "mentally ill" with its dominant, widespread representation. Therefore, a counter representation is timely, and so this politics of "people with lived experience". Ordinarily (we) "patients" have been represented by scholars, researchers, journalists, lawyers and caregivers while those with direct experience, silenced or marginalized as people whose testimonies are unreliable. "Being" is not the same as believing, and this point cannot be said enough. One can genuinely have malaria and all the symptoms of it, but believing you have malaria while having nothing to prove it, don't mean one suffers from malaria.

Suffice it to say when I refer to lived experience I refer to the above two experiences. The first is the experience of *believing to be a psychiatric patient* and therefore a subject of psychiatry. From that perspective emerges the idea of "narrative surrender" or becoming a *psychiatric subject*, not simply another "patient". The second experience plotted under the heading of recovery is not the recovery of the pathological in the person as though some "illness" has been cured, but recovering the "narrative", identity and sense of self.

Experience is a starting point and constituent of my politics: to prioritize certain voices over others and to analyse certain dominances in society by looking at psychiatry through a discursive lens, instead of a reductionist one. Neither is my politics identity based nor making an essentialist claim that the "mentally ill" constitute a particular kind of population whose representation I offer. In leveraging experience, my effort lies in analysing what peers shared with me by passing it through the analytical filters I utilize (Chapter 3).

Recovery and its politics

The roots of the idea of recovery go back into the 18th century,[2] yet an active engagement with the idea began to emerge with the work of psychiatric survivors, who started making efforts to support their peers by creating empathic, supportive and empowering services. When mainstream psychiatry recognized their viability, there was a move within psychiatry to bring recovery into mental health policies. In this co-option, of both the recovery idea and the peer's role, by psychiatry two things changed significantly. The first was the empowering role played by peers in supporting others'

2 At that time India was a British colony and there was no such development in India. I discuss this in greater detail in Chapter 6. Whatever historical antecedents I mention here belong largely to those countries of the Global North where "recovery" is already part of mental health policy.

recovery became dependent on psychiatric decisions; becoming *psychiatry-led*, not peer-assisted. The second change was in the *nature of recovery* itself; "treatment" and recovery were henceforth treated synonymously. This co-option creates challenges and complexity that merit scrutiny.

Upon receiving a diagnosis of "psychosis", everyone takes time to understand it: a stage wherein accepting the role of "patient" they make adjustments, exploring all options – both for recovery and healing. Everyone tries adapting for only by walking through the labyrinth recovery occurs. It takes time, prolonged adjustments, developing skills, knowledge and insight(s) into understanding one's life and its unique challenges.

Why is recovery so complicated it inspires polar opposite views and becomes politicized? What is the nature of such politics? Let us try refining the dilemma first. To recognize recovery, we have to agree there is recovery: something needs to be recovered from. This dovetails into an ontological question – whether one believes or not what needs to be recovered from, which here is "psychosis". What changes if we believe that "psychosis" is nothing but a diagnostic name given to overwhelming suffering vis-à-vis taking a perspective that "psychosis" is a real "disease" to be treated by pharmaceutical potions? This binary in conceptualizing "psychosis" as real/material versus a consensual truth, agreed upon by a group having interests in establishing it as such (see Bueter, 2019) indicates the category "psychosis" is contestable. Until pathology can be established by tests and measures, there cannot be recovery from the same.

My ontological position is that "mental illness" is *not* a material reality but socially constructed. This disparity is the first element of the politics of recovery – between those who wish to establish recovery as a *medical outcome* as opposed to those who wish to see it as a *reclamation project*. In other words, "psychosis" and recovery have biological versus sociological causality. In the biological idea, recovery lies via a medical regimen; in the latter, it emerges in the space of social justice and equity.

Nevertheless acknowledging suffering to be real and efforts to heal being outcomes of individual subjectivity recovery is approached, not by foisting on peers a contrasting ontological position: non-belief in "mental illness".[3] Davidson et al. (2010:5) remind that the possibility of people resolving their deep crises and suffering has been accepted from the days of the "moral treatment" when humane staff used gentle, supportive and primarily educational interventions to help the residents of their asylums get back on their feet and resume their normal routines and responsibilities, a time during which recovery rates were estimated to be as high as 90%.

---

3 Whoever arrives at this ontology has developed over time considerable critical ability to contest and challenge such a powerful institution as psychiatry currently is.

Divergences on recovery

Recovery as an idea does not evoke a unanimous response. The current ubiquity of the term recovery, alongside its vagueness, probably reflects a phase in high modernity of optimism and relativism (Pilgrim, 2008:295). Three broad views of recovery are prevalent currently, namely, (a) the psychiatric or biomedical view defining recovery from a clinical or curative orientation, (b) a community-based integration perspective adopted by social psychiatry, which talks about and extends the rehabilitation perspective and (c) an emancipatory view of those who have interacted with the psychiatric system and challenge coercive treatment regimens.

In this book, the focus lies on two poles: clinical and emancipatory views. Social psychiatry may be seen as a subset of the clinical view, or an amalgam of the two; for once someone becomes a "patient" they always work towards rehabilitation, which may/not lead to complete recovery. Thus, focusing on recovery I distinguish two ideas without digressing into sub-categories: either someone becomes drugs and symptom free or they remain drug dependent. In psychiatric terms, this is a difference between the phrases *"recovery in"* as though it is an ongoing process and *"recovery from"* which means recovery has been accomplished (Davidson and Roe, 2007). The "recovery from" idea is based upon recorded longitudinal evidence of people with diagnoses of severe mental illness becoming symptom free and not returning to the patient role (in Pilgrim, 2008:296). This might occur after one acute episode or years of episodic tumult. The "recovery in" notion is more of an ongoing effort to adjust with a "mental illness" and progressing in spite of a vulnerability of relapse or ongoing symptoms. I illustrate this difference in my analysis in Chapters 4 and 6. For now, I distinguish the manner "recovery" is conceptualized by two major stakeholders with opposing views, viz., psychiatrists and "ex-patients".

Recovery is not a sudden process of reclaiming self-hood for people who have been through the mental health system but a gradual change in the rehabilitation efforts they have been making. For most of us, recovery is not a sudden conversion experience. Hope does not come to us as a sudden bolt of lightning that jolts us into a whole new way of being. Hope is the turning point that must quickly be followed by the willingness to act (Deegan, 1988:14). Roe and Lachman (2005:226) emphasize the experience of self among people with schizophrenia, suggesting the individual's experience of self is a central theoretical construct in the understanding and treatment of schizophrenia and related disorders. The latter is psychiatry's view best exemplified as a "deeply personal, unique process of changing one's attitudes, values, feelings, goals, skills and/or roles. It is a way of living a satisfying, hopeful, and contributing life even with limitations caused by illness" (Anthony, 1993).

It would seem uncontroversial that recovery is possible and desirable and should be the main purpose of mental health services Wallcraft (2009) noted at the Critical Psychiatry Network Conference. Yet she bemoaned that psychiatric services often emphasize maintenance rather than recovery. While to Wallcraft recovery seems an obvious choice, for why else would a person agree to be "treated", to Anthony, who represents professional views, a life lived with the symptoms and ongoing treatment is just as good. There appears to be little need for drug-free recovery as long as the individual can remain functional with ongoing treatment!

Although standardized measures have contributed to the reliability of concepts[4] and improved communication, they have also hindered readiness to consider other potentially important phenomena. Roe and Lachman are critical of the manner in which psychiatry conceptualizes measures and studies mental illness.

> [A] narrow focus on symptoms and pathology has oversimplified the complexity of mental illness, leading to the false conception that the person afflicted by the illness is "entirely ill." As a result, little attention has been given to the possibility of simultaneous presence of strengths and weaknesses, competence and dysfunction. This has discouraged paying attention to the healthy and restored parts of the person and his or her experience of living and coping with a severe mental disorder.
>
> (Roe and Lachman, 2005:223)

This idea has implications from the point of view of recovery: it underscores rehabilitation. Someone considered "ill" is not altogether incapable of doing anything. The emphasis is for changing the thinking about "illness" itself while creating more opportunities for rehabilitation. Meanwhile, Harper and Speed (2012:8) characterize recovery as a "struggle for recognition", founded on a model of identity politics which displaces and marginalizes the need for social, political and economic redistribution to address many of the underlying causes of emotional distress. They propose this as the location where one could locate mental distress, instead of people's biological make-up. This view is close to the position taken by ex-patients.

It is visible that survivor or emancipatory perspectives have been co-opted by psychiatry, in the process obliterating the radical critique they offered against psychiatry. The model of recovery currently implemented in

---

4 While saying that standardized measures may map and measure certain aspects of "psychopathology" it was noted in the Chapter 1 the definitional issues of "psychosis" are not yet universally agreed upon. These claims of psychiatric professionals need to be taken somewhat cautiously.

many countries is a professional admixture of rehabilitation options guided by psychiatry. This is the reason why ongoing "patienthood" remains central to their notion of recovery.

Recovery movement in psychiatry

The current day recovery movement in psychiatry reflects the psychiatric survivor movement that started in the US in the 1970s and 1980s, having repercussions across the globe (Roberts and Boardman, 2013). The emergence of a large body of the literature by people who have been consumers of psychiatric services, in various parts of the world (Chamberlin, 1984; Deegan, 1988; Miller, 2008; Leamy et al., 2011; Sharma, 2011; Helman, 2017) attest the fact that recovery in mental health is a reality that can be accomplished by many.

The National Institute of Mental Health Recovery in England (in Slade and Hayward, 2007:81) defines recovery as a personal process of overcoming the negative impact of diagnosed mental illness/distress despite its continued presence. One branch of the recovery literature distinguishes between clinical and personal recovery (Davidson et al., 2005; Slade, 2010). For Roe et al. (2011:133), recovery may be broadly organized into two categories which have been labeled as objective versus subjective (Lysaker et al., 2006) or clinical versus personal (Slade et al., 2008). Resnick et al. (in Lysaker et al., 2006:223) propose recovery can involve changes in any of a number of domains of function that can be grouped into at least two larger sets: objective assessments of the absence of illness (e.g., symptom remission and good psychosocial function) and subjective experiences related to attitudes and/or life orientation (e.g., hopefulness). They suggest that in addition to life attitudes and orientation, the subjective domain of recovery can be conceptualized as including changes in qualities of self-experience.

The roots of the recovery movement in psychiatry have been traced back to humanistic philosophers, social activists and compassionate clinicians over the past couple of hundred years (Davidson in Roberts and Boardman, 2013:400). Davidson et al. (2010:9) also note that the primary challenge for recovery-oriented practice is how to educate, encourage and support people with serious mental illnesses as they go about trying to figure out how to live a meaningful life with, compensate for and perhaps eventually overcome a serious mental illness. Liberman and Kopelowicz (2005:735) distinguish ideas of recovery as a process versus outcome of recovery. They propose that the process and stages of recovering are preparations for recovery. Characterized by a reliable normative definition, recovery is an outcome of the process of recovering. Individuals can take many pathways to recovery depending on the varied factors that influence the process, such as personal attributes, social environment, continuity and quality of treatment, and subjective experiences.

In the historical development of the idea of recovery, heterogeneity was discovered in the course and outcome of illnesses across people, as also across various domains of functioning within any given individual and over time (Davidson and Roe, 2007:461) Researchers discovered that "mental illnesses" were multi-dimensional disorders composed of several domains of functioning which were both conceptually and empirically distinct. People were seen to be recovering in some domains of life, including in living independently, taking up employment while experiencing impairments in other domains of life, such as psychotic symptoms or hearing voices. Various descriptions such as concepts of symptomatic recovery, partial recovery and social recovery began to be used to describe various outcomes.

How does recovery occur?

Recovery is ideologically associated with wellness (Cummings and Bentley, 2018), grounded in principles of self-determination, hope for change and mutual support. The above segment inaugurates the distinction between recovery the way ex-/patients as opposed to psychiatry visualize it; both differ from each another, as also in the means adopted to recover. In Szasz's referral to human interests, at the start of this chapter, there is a reminder that humans act in accordance with their self-interest: each must know her own.

For Borg (2007:5), recovery means taking back control and getting on with one's life, managing most things most of the time, albeit in one's own ways or at one's own pace. Recovery is not about cure nor necessarily about symptom eradication, but rather about learning to live with and gaining more control over what is distressful. This psy-professionals' perspective accepts recovery as a fluid, ambivalent concept having subjective variations. Yet even though similar views are prevalent for almost two decades in many countries of the Global North due to policy prescriptions, mainstream recovery initiatives have come under criticism in these countries.

Recovery has been implemented as a policy measure in many countries, especially Australia, the US, UK and Japan (see Sharma, 2019), keeping peers at the forefront. Here mainstream psychiatric clinics involve peers in small, supportive roles; as adjuncts supporting psychiatric goals, for such systems largely work under the guidance of psychiatrists. This co-optation of recovery does not necessarily empower patients, instead facilitating the uptake of medication by more people, with lesser resistance. Due to this lopsidedness and lack of clarity about its meaning or outcomes, the idea and implementation of the recovery model have come under severe criticism. In the context of Britain, Pilgrim (2008:296) notes that any enthusiasm for, or true commitment to, recovery or "care in the community" is constantly tempered by anxiety about risk, from any party constructing and enacting mental health policy. Harper and Speed (2012:9–10) problematize the manner in which recovery and resilience are depicted as a uniformly positive development in the mental health field. They are critical of the rise of recovery phenomenon for three reasons: (a) it is an individualistic, neoliberal identity politics of certain people not based on redistributive justice; (b) it reflects a failure to challenge the underlying deficit based understanding of people; and (c) it ignores structural factors of health and social inequalities.

From a social justice orientation, Morrow and Weisser (2012:28) advocate for centralizing the profound discrimination faced by people who have been psychiatrized and the connections between recovery and the social and structural barriers that shape, facilitate or impede recovery. These social and structural aspects are articulated and enacted through a number of dimensions of power such as biomedicalism, racialization, sanism, sexism, ageism, heterosexismand more , necessitating an intersectional social justice analysis of recovery. Seen from "patient" and professional perspectives, recovery has different hues and no analysis of barriers to recovery can be complete without examining the structural barriers the individual "patient" faces.

Recovery and the Indian context

Indian policymakers have been showing interest in the idea of recovery for the last few years in response to the developments in the Global North. The earliest reference to recovery is visible in the Mental Healthcare Bill of 2013, when there was a talk of repealing the Mental Health Act of 1987. The bill proposed that "[p]ersons with mental illness should be treated like other persons with health problems and the environment around them should be made conducive to facilitate recovery, rehabilitation and full participation in society" (MoHFW:56). Soon after in 2014, the ministry released a policy document titled *New Pathways, New Hope* in which they defined recovery as "a process of change through which individuals improve their health and wellbeing, live a self-directed life and strive to reach their full potential" (MoHFW, 2014:i). Rao (2015:S2) speaking at the 67th Annual conference of Indian Psychiatric Society with the theme of "Mental Illness – Recovery & Social Inclusiveness" noted about advances of psychopharmacology, clinical psychology, neuro-psychology, modern behaviour therapies claiming due to these developments we are able to bring superior changes in our patients' recovery from their sufferings (Rao, 2015:S2). In minuscule ways, the idea of recovery is gaining visibility in the Indian policy and linguistic landscape, albeit in a rhetorical, normative manner, mostly conflating "treatment gap" with recovery. Its main premise is that since people have limited access to psychiatric services, *once they have the requisite access, their treatment goals are automatically met*!

Bayetti et al. (2016:889) question the zeal to implement a Global North inspired "Recovery Model" in India. They propose "a fundamental rethinking of existing culturally incongruent 'Recovery Models' before application in India's public mental health and clinic settings". In Chapter 6, I continue further with other conceptual, social justice and ontological issues that reflect upon the viability of recovery in the Indian society.

Personal aspects of "recovery"

True recovery, says Helman (2017:2) is essentially the same as remission, but with two major difference – (a) symptoms are no longer managed by medication, and (b) those symptoms are no longer active. Just as most of the population is free from a sense of impending crisis, so too, the recovered "mental patient" is free. There are several key enablers to "recovery", such as employment, inclusion in community, independent living, significant relationships, etc. Psychotherapy with a supportive therapist has been cited as a positive contributor to recovery (Bjornestad et al., 2018).

Liberman and Kopelowicz (2005:735) enlist attributes of individuals who are progressing toward recovery as hope, destigmatization, empowerment, self-acceptance, insight, awareness, collaboration with professionals, sense of autonomy and self-control, and participation in self-help and consumer-run programs. While these authors also hint at remaining compliant to professional views, I delve into some of these to understand their role in supporting, establishing and consolidating recoveries of my research contributors in Chapters 4 and 5.

My views about recovery

From discussions with contributors to this study and their caregivers, personal patienthood, delving into literature, there is little ambiguity recovery refers to leaving behind a psychiatric past, including being medicated against one's wishes. Whether someone has given up medical dependence or not, they count the ending of medication as the real yardstick to measure recovery. Psychiatrists may view recovery as a personal journey even with ongoing medication but that is their professional view. For current and past "patients", the challenge is always to exit pharmacological treatments. In countries where the recovery model exists as the goal of the mental health treatments, drug-assisted recovery is taken as the norm.

Definitional debates about recovery reflect wider ideological debates about the nature of mental health (Harper and Speed, 2012:8) being a crucial starting point. For here, which marks the beginning, there exists an ontological divergence between (at least some) stakeholders.

Recovery, as I see, is a complex set of individual efforts embedded within a social-relational process, vitally dependent upon how people are supported by their environment to accomplish life goals affirming their worth, abilities and capabilities. Inasmuch as anyone has a right to define their suffering, whether "illness" or a passing phase, everyone also has a right to choose recovery over non-recovery or going off medication versus continuing taking medication. I formulate my idea of recovery starting from the position taken by the early psychiatric survivors, Judi Chamberlin[5] and Pat Deegan.[6]

It is a two-stage process: (a) beyond patienthood, accompanied by an end of dependence on medication, (b) emergence of a knowledge orientation which enables someone to recover their self-hood from the domination of a culturally established and agreed upon "vocabulary of psychological deficit" (Gergen, 1997:147), standardized and propagated by mainstream psychiatry. In sum, I conceptualize "recovery" as a change in the world-view one has become accustomed to: moving away from "mental illness", and evolving new ideas, tools and understandings to deal with day-to-day challenges without spiralling into a breakdown.

Being knower: epistemic violence and its consequences

While lived experience may be a starting point one needs to question whose knowledge matters? Can people who have been "patients" stake an epistemic claim? Here, the idea of epistemic violence, endemic to the field of mental health, becomes operative. "Epistemic" represents the idea of knowledge and its construction. Which person or social groups can be legitimate contributors to knowledge construction?

In contemporary society, certain groups exist whose knowledge is considered valuable, trustworthy and relevant as opposed to others who do not evoke such trust. Gayatri Spivak uses the term *epistemic violence* in her text, "Can the Subaltern Speak?" as a way of marking the silencing of marginalized groups (Dotson, 2011:236).

An example of the same from Liegghio (2013) illustrates the case for "mental illness". Speaking in the context of her mother's experience of dying of cancer yet forced to be in a palliative care unit for psychiatric patients against her wishes she is anguished about a system where the psychiatrized people are routinely denied their personhood due to an endemic and routinized form of violence, called epistemic violence (Spivak, 1988:24). Even though her mother did not want to be in hospital, yet someone who was going through her case papers discovered that she had been diagnosed with a "mental illness" in the past and decided she was best off staying in hospital. So they took away the state support she was offered in her home and forced

---

5 Most psychiatrists seem to think that a little psychiatry would be good for everyone, and that not knowing that you are "ill" is one of the "symptoms" of the "illness", and so people need to be coerced. But this is not the way things are supposed to work in a free society (Chamberlin, 1998:406).

6 The goal is to embrace our human vocation of becoming more deeply, more fully human (Deegan, 1996:92).

her to move into palliative care. Epistemic violence refers to the way certain persons or groups within society are disqualified as legitimate knowers at a structural level through various institutional processes and practices. For an individual to be disqualified as a legitimate knower, certain constructions become necessary in order to justify the disqualification. For psychiatrized people, being constructed as "incompetent" and "dangerous" becomes a powerful mechanism leading to their disqualification as legitimate knowers (Liegghio, 2013:125).

By denying people the right to represent their truth and invalidating what they say, there is an injustice committed against them. Fricker (2007:1) proposes the idea of epistemic injustice as a wrong done to someone specifically in their capacity as a knower. She distinguishes between two kinds of epistemic injustice, viz., testimonial and hermeneutical injustice. "Testimonial injustice occurs when prejudice causes a hearer to give a deflated level of credibility to a speaker's word; hermeneutical injustice occurs at a prior stage, when a gap in collective interpretive resources puts someone at an unfair disadvantage when it comes to making sense of their social experiences" (Fricker, 2007:1). Hermeneutical injustice implies that since people do not know how to interpret what someone is saying, they do not give credibility to their testimony and even before hearing them fully, they may dismiss their point of view or experience. This idea has important consequences for those with "mental illness" labels because their testimonies are regularly dismissed, for people do not wish to engage with them independently. This study attempts to address this issue specifically – by centralizing the testimonies of those given diagnosis and analyzing their narratives, illustrating how this marginalization occurs all the time.

There are two other interlinked ideas proposed by Fricker consistent with this study, namely, social power and identity power. She defines power as a socially situated capacity to control others' actions (Fricker, 2007:4) and then introduces a new subspecies of social power, calling it *identity power*. This phrase implies that some identities will automatically inspire more power, confidence and faith in their ideas and some will suffer from a deficit on those counts, because of what she terms as *identity prejudice*[7] – a label for prejudices against people *qua* social type. Naturally enough, those who have social power will also enjoy an identity power, and those who suffer from an identity deficit will not enjoy a similar kind of social power. Reconfiguring this in terms of epistemic claims, Carel and Kidd (2014:530) suggest the idea of epistemic privilege or that health professionals are considered to be epistemically privileged, in both warranted and unwarranted ways, by virtue of their training, expertise and third person psychology.

---

7 Italics original.

The "mentally ill" person distinctly suffers from an identity prejudice for they are not only undermined in their capacity as knowers, or representatives of their truth but due to pre-existing diagnostic categories into which their storied accounts can be readily interpreted and re-storied; their experiences do not get validated as suffering, getting slotted instead as "illness". It is noteworthy "how power differentials shape the status and recognition of different knowledge systems" (Jovchelovich, 2008:24). In this case, the power of psychiatry is much more than the power that "patients" have or can lay claim to. If individuals in both groups represent views about "patients", it is very likely that the claim of psychiatrists will be accorded greater salience than the representation of "patients" themselves. Of course, the fact that psychiatrists may be seen as a coherent group, whereas "patients" often do not constitute a group in such an organized manner contributes to this dominance in no small measure.

Usually, anything said by a person given a diagnosis is suspect and considered unreliable because they are attributed a certain inability to "understand reality" in a proper way. This constitutes *testimonial injustice*. Carel and Kidd (2014:531) give further evidence of epistemic injustice in healthcare in general and suggest that an ill person may be regarded as cognitively unreliable, emotionally compromised, existentially unstable or otherwise epistemically unreliable in a way that renders their testimonies and interpretations suspect simply by virtue of their status as an ill person with little sensitivity to their factual condition and state of mind.

Any epistemic injustice wrongs someone in their capacity as a subject of knowledge, and thus in a capacity essential to human value; and the particular way in which testimonial injustice does this is that a hearer wrongs a speaker in his capacity as a giver of knowledge, as an informant (Fricker, 2007:5). Fricker further argues that the primary harm one incurs in being wronged in this way is an intrinsic injustice, which may go into the psychology of the subject, and cramp self-development, so they may be quite literally prevented from becoming who they are. Lives of psychiatrized people largely unfold along this template. Therefore, a philosophical belief that people not be treated as mere subjects of inquiry by others but recognized as intelligent, responsive and trustworthy is the core epistemic belief towards which this book converges from diverse directions. In recognizing those given mental "illness" diagnosis as one such group, and bringing forth their knowledge via their unmediated, unsupervised testimonies, the goal is to challenge this historical silencing at least in some way.

I do not believe that people given mental "illness" diagnosis do not understand their reality or cannot represent their distress appropriately. I am convinced those who have experience understand at least their own experience better than anyone who can represent it. For me, this becomes an opportunity to hear their constructions, instead of psychiatric constructions about them is an act of "restoring a person's epistemic existence ... and give legitimacy to the person as someone with legitimate ways of knowing and, ultimately, legitimate ways of being" (Liegghio, 2013:127).

Dorothy Smith (in Liegghio, 2013:124) proposes that "mental illness" is a social construction formed at the place where people's experiences intersect with psychiatry – its structures and practices. This is the location where exists a possibility for psychiatry to take over the idea of the person's reality and self while creating a scope for them to become a psychiatric "patient". This sets into motion another complex process: subjectivation.

Subjecthood and subjectivation

The French theorist Michel Foucault has contributed significant ideas to current discussions about the nature, existence and exercise of power within contemporary mental health care (Roberts, 2005:33). He emphasized upon the relationship between power and knowledge, especially in the context of mental health. Knowledge and power are central to the process by which people are "made subjects" and therefore how psychiatric identities are produced (Roberts, 2005:33–34). In fact, towards the end of his life, Foucault considered subjectivation so significant he remarked the primary objective of his work had been to give a history of the different ways in which, throughout Western cultures, "human beings are made subjects" (Roberts, 2005:34). To comprehend subjectivation, it may be relevant to examine a linked idea: governmentality, which involves "governing the self" and "governing others" (Lemke, 2002:49).

Foucault examines government as both a practice and a problematic that first emerges in the 16th century, as a general problem dispersed across quite different areas of life, coining the term "governmentality" as a neologism for government rationality, one that links both "govern" and "mentality" (Besley, 2010:530). Foucault (in Besley, 2010) notes that governmentality means the complex of calculations, programmes, policies, strategies, reflections, and tactics that shape the conduct of individuals, "the conduct of conduct" for acting upon the actions of others in order to achieve certain ends.

In the context of this research, individuals who merit this governance are the "patients", having entered the ranks of the governable due to their diagnosis.[8] Governmentality in mental health would imply the manner in which policies are created to govern the conduct of people who are identified as needing the services of psy-professions. Governing "patients" requires a com-

---

8 This can be seen on a continuum mentioned by Goffman (1961) in *Asylums*, wherein certain groups are isolated and incarcerated, in what he calls *total* institutions where all persons of a certain kind are kept together for the sake of governing them. They are away from society for they are seen as a threat to societal functioning. Historically the "mentally ill" have been among these groups equally as much as other prison populations.

plex process, which is set in motion at the policy level where it is decided how "such" people may be treated in society – whether they be put outside the city as it was from the 19th century, be kept behind close walls in asylums or live in the community with families. Apart from this in what manner can these people be treated – by biochemical means, by therapies of various kinds, by complementary and alternatives practices like *ayurveda* or homeopathy and what would their civil, political, economic rights be. The whole cornucopia of these issues would amount to governing the citizens identified as "patients".

But what may happen with other "patients" takes a different form when it comes to psychiatry. As I have mentioned earlier, psychiatric patients often suffer from an identity prejudice and their testimonies about themselves are considered unreliable. Even if they speak, their accounts are dismissed or marginalized. Ordinarily, they do not enjoy the epistemic validity of any other citizen and portrayed incapable of representing themselves. This implies that they become subjects of governance who require monitoring, control and accountability.

If one were to suggest that psychiatric "patients" are individuals who need to be taken care of (or governed) by certain mechanisms, someone has to be in authority of that governance – lay down rules by which these "subjects" would be identified, classified and then monitored. This subject formation happens due to the presence of the institution of psychiatry – which lays down rules of behaviour and what classifies as normal versus what may be seen abnormal. "[T]he diagnostic and therapeutic practices of contemporary mental health care rest upon, and are informed by, a "body of psychiatric knowledge" (Roberts, 2005:37). Psychiatry has assumed the power to define for the whole society what may be considered as "acceptable" behaviour. The basis of this power lies in the claim to knowledge that psychiatry enjoys – for it has the explanatory capacity to explain the behaviours of those it observes, whereas those whose behaviours are being defined do not have such an explanatory capacity. This power-knowledge interplay establishes psychiatric power, making patients as "subjects", who lose their ability to be accepted as people with a viable point of view,and who need to be managed, governed and guided in most aspects of life henceforth.

What or who is taken to the "expert" in search of a solution? How does the layperson's story become identified with a diagnostic label? What happens to someone and their self-narrative when they become a subject of psychiatry? Where goes the original story which they had come and what ensues agreeable enough for the "patient" to embrace the label? To understand this we next look at ...

Narrative surrender

Sociologist Arthur Frank (1997) remarks that the modern experience of medicine begins when popular experience is overtaken by technical expertise. People go to experts who have their well-defined language and expressions for what the "patients" bring to them as their stories. Paid professionals now re-interpret their pains as symptoms, using a specialized language that is unfamiliar and overwhelming (Frank, 1997:5). This process in which one person's language and expression is changed into a new, medical version opens up the scope for those diagnosed taking on the "sick role", a phrase suggested by Talcott Parsons. He proposes that a core social expectation of being sick is surrendering oneself to the care of a physician. Frank on the other hand calls this process *narrative surrender* and marks it as a central moment in modernist illness experience. "The ill person not only agrees to follow physical regimens that are prescribed; she also agrees, tacitly but with no less implication, to tell her story in medical terms" (Frank, 1997:6).

This process, of the lay narrative transforming into the medical narrative, which is conveyed back to the person who reports the distress initially, and its adoption by her, to henceforth assume the role of the "patient" is one of the key aspects of modernist medicine. The exercise is accomplished by a complex coalition of several other factors, which I have explained in various segments of this framework. I illustrate the process of this transformation more fully in my analysis-based Chapters 4 and 5.

The constructed nature of reality

The fundamental idea underlying social construction is that the world is our construction (Gergen and Gergen, 2008:8). Simple as it may appear, the implications of this foundational idea are vast. "*Nothing*[9] is real unless people agree that it is" (ibid:10). Social construction inquiry is based on explicating the processes by which people make sense of the world they live in, including themselves according to Gergen (1985). As an approach to the social sciences, it draws its influences from a number of disciplines, including philosophy, sociology and linguistics (Burr, 2003:2). While explaining this at a theoretical level, Burr (2003) elaborates that a social constructionist orientation rests on one or more of the following assumptions (a) radical doubt in the taken for granted world (ibid: 267); (b) the world is constructed based on a historical and cultural bases (ibid:267); (c) historical and cultural specificity, which implies that all ways of understanding are historically and culturally relative (ibid: 3–4); (d) knowledge is an outcome of social processes between people, and is constantly negotiated, rather than having a fixed permanent finality.

Constructionists invite a dialogue around these ideas as a ground for further engagement between people, and to challenge the commonly held

---

9 Authors' original emphasis.

assumptions of what is constituted as "truth", "reality" or "knowledge". For constructionists, actions are not constrained by anything traditionally accepted as true, rational or right (ibid:12). I have adopted this attitude towards this book, and further invite the reader into this dialogue: to comprehend my goals and engage with understanding recovery from "psychosis", in an Indian milieu. I began from the start of everyone's narrative of "mental illness", which took me from the early roots of their suffering to later struggles to rehabilitate or recover. The latter are also socially constructed and I trace their pathways inasmuch as I first cast a theoretical glance at them.

Having believed myself to be a "patient" for nearly two decades making a switch in conception of mental "illness" from a disease/illness orientation to a social construction was by far the most difficult personal and ontological challenge I encountered. But once the nudge for reframing occurred, it also became the start of my story of research in it. This occurred due to a chance encounter with social constructionist theory, beginning at the start of the decade 2010–2011. What began as an attempt to understand my personal recovery in time pushed me to extend the inquiry towards others. At the earliest stages itself and contrary to what I had believed earlier, "mental illnesses are no longer limited to the personal histories of individuals alone but can also be seen as illnesses whose trigger could have come from the communal sphere" (Sharma, 2011:189). Until then, like others I also believed that a "mental illness" was a biological truth and there was something a medical intervention would resolve, bring healing. Encountering constructionism led me to the question – what if "mental illness" was a construction, and the roots of the "illness" did not lie in the person at all, but somewhere outside? So the challenge after my narrative became that I would have to examine more narratives similarly.

But whereas in a personal narrative, all biographical facts are known for another's, the same analysis cannot just be a straightforward application of pre-set criteria. An examination of many factors is required to draw a conclusive picture, gaining clarity whether a flow of events and similar tropes become apparent across narratives. In every narrative a social construction of "illness" or "recovery" becomes visible. From my story, I could only see the socially constructed nature of my "illness" and recovery, but to examine the phenomena as a wider reality necessitated a thorough, reflexive search to prove that indeed the construction of "mental illness" occurs across stories.

This necessitates an exposition of the philosophical premises of social construction and why I settled for it as the meta-theoretical framework for this book.

Emergence of social construction

In his earliest struggles to understand the social nature of knowledge, Gergen (1996) notes his uneasiness with social psychology as it was dedicated to predicting and understanding social behaviour, which in itself is inherently unstable. He took two ideas, one each from Gadamer and Thomas Kuhn both of who seemed to be pointing in a similar direction. Gadamer was grappling with the hermeneutical dilemma of how the meaning of a text is interpreted by a reader. Kuhn meanwhile had demonstrated the ways in which the interpretation of scientific evidence is largely guided by a paradigm of understanding (or theoretical forestructure) central to the field at any given time. As he reasoned, the scientist carries out research and interprets the findings in terms of a theoretical (and metatheoretical) framework (or set of a priori assumptions) shared within a particular community. An identical conclusion via literary theory was reached by Stanley Fish who showed that "when readers attempt to understand a text, they do so as members of an interpretive community. Their interpretations will inevitably bear the conventional understandings of the community" (Gergen, 1996). From diverse directions, one idea began to appear clearly: people make sense of events within a certain set of understandings, which they collectively agree upon.

Gergen (1996) further notes that social construction oriented social psychologists started looking in other directions for research, away from traditional human experimentation, to explore the ways in which reality is constructed within society. The chief way to conduct these studies was by focusing on language, as the earlier paragraph indicated, the interpretive tool within communities.

> These studies, which focus on the discursive means by which we determine what is true and good, are emancipatory in their aims. Rather than trying to demonstrate universal principles, they use discourse analysis to foreground our particular habits of constructing the world and ourselves.

The reality that concerns this book is the reality of "mental illness", and social constructionism assists here to examine the basis of this "reality". The claim to truth of this "reality" is complicated by the fact that though mental "illness" is said to exist within people, its existence cannot be established by any objective means. This implies that the basis of this existence is solely dependent upon the interpretive or representational capacity of the "expert" who classifies any apparent or visibly disturbed behaviour as "illness". Since there is nothing to be determined by any objectives tests or measures, the only means left to establish the presence of a "mental illness" is language. At the first level, it is the language in which the "patient" narrates her distress to the "expert" and at the next a metamorphosis of this (lay) narration into the expert's technical language. The capacity lies with the expert, not the lay person; they only have a claim to the expression, no control over how it would be interpreted.

Gergen (1997:34) draws attention to the struggle that both scientists and empiricist philosophers have waged for decades now, "to remove the sciences from moral debate". In their search for an objective, value neutral science they have tried to focus on "what is the case", instead of "what ought to be", the latter being viewed as not being a scientific concern. Gergen writes that the principal ideological critique for the empiricism and rationality which emerged with the Enlightenment began to be questioned during moral outrage that accompanied the Vietnam war. Social scientists then began to question the moral neutrality of the sciences in perpetrating an imperious brutality and further efforts by the scientific establishment to enhancing the technologies of aggression. It was this disaffection with the commitment to positivist philosophy of science, capitalism and bourgeois liberalism, which had ushered in "such evils as erosion of community, the deterioration of moral values, the establishment of dominance relationships" (Gergen, 1997:34) that led to the rise of "critical theory", having a goal of ideological emancipation. The purpose of critical theory was to question the premise of Enlightenment rationality and its consequent impact on humans, relationships and the ecology. "Critical appraisal thus liberates us from the pernicious effects of mystifying truths" (Gergen, 1997:35). It is in this spirit that I approach this inquiry: questioning the self-evident basis of *truth* of psychiatric diagnosis, the morality of psychiatric treatment and comprehending the impact of psychiatric dominance on recovery outcomes from "psychosis".

Knowledge as social construction

Gergen draws attention to the social nature of knowledge, rather than the rational individualism proposed by Enlightenment. For Ian Hacking a primary use of "social construction" has been for raising consciousness. This is done in two distinct ways, one overarching the other more localized (1999:6). So while all experience may be construed as socially constructed, at a local level, one talks of a specific experience. For instance, the experiences of caste, marriage and toothache are socially constructed among people who agree upon the meaning these words conjure, for they carry a culturally accepted meaning. Local claims are in principle independent of each other. A person may be a social constructionist on the theme of the caste system or female foeticide yet believe that mental illness is real!

Until the arrival of social construction, the socio-behavioral sciences have traditionally been trying to render objective accounts of human conduct and to explain its character in a universal manner. But how realistic can such an objective representation be since language may not always be able to "depict, mirror, contain, convey or store objective knowledge" (Gergen, 1997:33). Is there knowledge outside of a relational context, embedded in a social matrix? The notion of individual knowledge gained in solitude is replaced by "a view of knowledge as lodged within the sphere of social re-latedness" (Gergen, 1997:30).

How do communities that share common cultural understandings con-struct its meaning? Is it because of shared symbols or syntactic structures? Social construction centralizes the role of language in understanding and constructing the world. Until we can speak the same language as someone, we cannot communicate with them as cultural equals. Yet, since language is also one of the important areas of my work, I defer its discussion to an-other location, while focusing on discourse here.

The key role of language is to make sense of our world, express experience and convey common understandings of reality as someone comprehends them. But what happens if experience is narrated in one language, trans-lated into another and then acted upon? In modern medicines, this pathway is taken by all patients in an attempt to convey their distress to doctors. Doctors then translate these experiential realities as signs and symptoms in terms of their pre-existing medical knowledge. Once the patient's narration is over, the doctor takes over the narrative and re-interprets it in terms of their own medical and diagnostic language. Whatever emerges from this re-interpretation is what the patient accepts as a medical truth, without verifying it in most cases. Ultimately, it comes to the point that the decision of how to deal with a patient's suffering is a matter of medical percep-tion. Foucault refers to this as the "sovereign power of the empirical gaze" (Foucault, 2003: xiii).

"Mental illness": a socially constructed discourse

By far, the most interesting aspect I found was the manner in which so-cial constructionists view "mental illness". Constructionist scholars have launched serious critiques against the taken-for-granted character of many social phenomenon such as suicide, beliefs, schizophrenia, altruism, etc. (Gergen, 1985:267). Their challenge to the objectivity-claim of "mental illness" as a socially constructed reality, instead of an objective reality piqued my curiosity to examine both "mental illness" and social construc-tion in equal measures. Deriving from the idea that knowledge is not an objective truth or reality, but a socially constructed understanding among people who share a cultural context, one can see the existence of "mental illness" as a consensual reality. The cultural context referred here is the training and education that psychiatrists undergo, which assists them de-velop a perception or "gaze" and ability to abstract diagnostic categories from lay accounts of people's distress.

Since construction of ideas occurs linguistically, language and its study becomes central to social construction. This is a time when biomedical and otherwise reductionist explanations and understandings of mental disorder are dominant in scholarly, scientific and psychotherapeutic worldviews and

51

practices (Fee, 2000:1). Fee establishes how "mental illness" is viewed – an unquestioned finality, an ontological certainty. Time and again constructionist scholars return to the theme of "mental illness" and question whether or how diagnostic labels assist someone in distress. Gergen (1997:143) goes further saying there is a reason to believe that in their very effort to furnish effective means of alleviating human suffering, mental health professionals simultaneously generate a network of increasing entanglements for the culture at large. Such entanglements are not only self-serving for the professions, they also add exponentially to the sense of human misery.

Considering "mental illness" is not measurable by any means, and is purely a matter of someone's understanding or observation, Hacking (1999: 100) also calls it a social construct. All communications which talk and represent "mental illness" never seem to question its basis; whether it a reality at all. Gergen (1997:147) says, "the prevailing ontology of mental life remains generally unchallenged". Constructionist inquiry is precisely about this – to examine the ontological basis of "mental illness", examine the discourse that represents "mental illness" and question its utility. When claims to truth are understood as social constructions, significant questions are opened on whose truth is given priority, who is silenced, who gains by the dominant discourse and who loses, and what ideologies and societal practices are sustained by the taken for granted realties (Sugiman et al., 2008:4). Discourse is a key theme social constructionist inquiry focuses on. Constructionists see it as the existence of culturally constructed meanings of phenomenon, among people who belong to communities. The nature of discourse comes under intense scrutiny and also constitutes the methodological choice for this book.

The nature of this inquiry is critical analysis – both in observing the occurrence of "illness" and recovery by those previously under the remit of psychiatry. So though social construction had tremendous appeal for those previously marginalized by science, and those in pursuits of social equality and justice, social constructionist progress has not altogether been unproblematic. Due to the discursive shift that social construction has emerged from, the door to broadscale political and moral critique of existing authority structure has become so prevalent that "societal conflict has become an increasingly commanding feature of the contemporary cultural landscape" (Gergen, 1998:148). If everything is a social construction, then how does one deal with suffering identified as "mental illness"? Can one take the path of rejecting the psychiatric alternative entirely? I attempt a response to this question at the end (Chapter 7). In Chapter 4, my focus is how someone's suffering is socially transformed to a diagnostic category.

Human sciences "mental health" research in India

Mental health research has been done by diverse scholars in the Indian context. My focus here is on social or human science research with emphasis on ethnographic evidence since that appears to be the method adopted by a majority of researchers. Nunley (1996, 1998) reports about ethnographic observations from two hospitals in North India to understand professional practices of psychiatrists in India and then a comparable evidence from the United States. Das and Addlakha (2001) explore notions of impairment and disability in two locations in Delhi, through a reconfiguration of the domestic sphere, whereas Addlakha (2008) focuses on the family and psychiatry in her ethnographic study of a hospital in Delhi. More ethnographic evidence comes from Kerala studied by Bindhulakshmi's (2006) ethnographic exploration into the lives of women and the social worlds in which they are engaged, Ranganathan (2011) studies spirit possession in the Mahanubhav temples of Maharashtra, Pinto (2013) analyses in-patient confinement in a female ward of a private psychiatric clinic in a north Indian city, and Sood (2016) in Balaji temple in Mehndipur, Rajasthan. Sousa (2016) examines the concept of diagnostic neutrality in Lucknow, Marrow (2016) investigates the role of marriage in transitions that women make in Varanasi, and Luhrmann and Padmavati (2016) report about schizophrenia from Chennai. Bayetti, Jadhav and Deshpande (2017) examine the training of psychiatrists in India via their clinical ethnographies. While Mathais investigates the impact of social exclusion on those with mental health diagnoses (2015), and individual and/or caregivers' narratives in Uttarakhand (2016), she also studies the impact of stigma and social distance people maintain from those given mental illness diagnoses (2018).

Closest to this study

Among all the above studies, the ones that seem closest to my work are ethnographic research studies by Bindhulakshmi (2006) and Addlakha (2008), carried out in Kerala and Delhi, respectively, among women and their families. All of us interviewed both "patients" and caregivers in our respective studies, yet there are significant divergences between us:

Ontology – While Addlakha's work begins with an ontological position relying on "mental illness" as a social category, Bindhulakshmi rejects "mental illness" as a material, objective reality, having a less definitive stance about the diagnostic "truth" it represents. Both researchers have studied the social worlds their informants inhabit. They have interviewed several actors in these milieus, which include professionals, family caregivers and "patients" themselves. They have gathered data originating from psychiatric hospital/clinic settings, as well as visited the homes of some of their research informants.

I take "mental illness" to be a social representation due to an interest group's power–knowledge claim. Philosophically, I reject "mental illness" as *reality*. It is but a subjective claim, which becomes hegemonic due to its close alignment with institutional mechanisms which can ensure its salience. There is some compatibility between Bindhulakshmi and my views here.

Position of researchers – These researchers are sociologists/ anthropologists, whereas I conduct my research as a peer, with the hindsight of experiencing "patienthood" and the psychiatric system. For me testimonies offered by peers are not only viable and truthful, but being part of my experience confirm that such experiences were not confined to either them or me; they are widely prevalent.

Whose representation – Both their studies include psychiatric points of view, while this book does not, focusing instead on "patient" and caregivers alone. Being a peer, my goals and methods are emancipatory and involve an attempt to restore the epistemic credibility of peers. For Addlakha and Bindhulakshmi, it appears a challenge to believe "patient" perspectives and they know not what a "psychotic" episode feels like. Therefore, it may be difficult for them to rely on testimonies[10] of their research informants alone; possibly they are unsure of their reliability.[11] They feel the need to rely on professional and caregivers' views more than I do, as the credibility we attribute to our respective informants' testimonies come from different experiential and epistemic perspectives.

Goals of study – Our respective goals are also different: they seek an explanation for "mental illness" among specific groups, I a pathway for recovery among peers. My research is predicated on the assumption that people can recover, while something holds them back from recovery, whilst these researchers are not examining this issue. They focus on their day-to-day struggles, challenges and realities. I know such realities myself and therefore there is little need to know them further. It is more pertinent to search for that which I do not know already – the barriers to recovery. Their goals are interpretive, mine emancipatory, accordingly our methods.

Research as future forming – My research has a "future forming" orientation (see Chapter 1), whereas Bindhulakshmi focuses on "giving primacy to the experiences of women diagnosed with mental illness" (2006) and attempts to understand the everyday tactics they use to fit into the "normal" world in which they live. Addlakha (2008:5) strives to show the complex interweaving of illness and culture in the context of mental disorder, to tell stories of the "mentally ill" in their own voices.

Our positions as researchers, starting points, epistemic positions, ontological assumptions and methods are different. My work may be seen as advancing the field of survivor research within and as part of Mad Studies,

---

10 I discuss about this in greater detail in the context of hermeneutical injustice.
11 This is not to imply that they do not have empathy with their research informants, for they come across as seasoned researchers working with a respectful stance. I say this to highlight the difference between knowing something from experience as opposed to knowing something from a cognitive, theoretical position.

and enriching it from the point of view of people who speak from experi-ence, in the spirit of *"nothing about us, without us"*. But there are other trajectories as well – in decoloniality, Mad Studies, law and policy reform and more.

This chapter created the framework of this book elaborating on its reasons, defining the sensibilities with which I approached my research questions and peers. I began with lived experience but do not believe that experience alone constitutes knowledge, therefore qualify the meaning of "experience" further. Thereafter, recovery is explained in its diverse defini-tions unraveling how help seeking leads to patienthood and unknowingly towards subjecthood. There are epistemic dis/advantages for certain groups in society. There exists a link between marginalization of people due to their de-valued identities; their testimonies are overshadowed by views of the epistemically dominant. The next chapter details the actual tasks of this book: meeting peers, listening to them, working through ethical and methodological challenges, and choosing tools to analyse their narratives.

3

AMONG PEERS, WHERE
ONE IS HOME

I am on my way. Start walking on the straight road from the intersection, I am coming towards you in a grey car, bearing this number.

I say to Nithya

I was waiting and she called, nearly there. She was coming to meet me from Delhi, the second peer to visit me. Rupali, the first had dropped in a few days earlier and since we knew one another for years, it was easier to assimilate her narrative prior to meeting an unknown person. Interviewing Rupali also helped zero in on pertinent questions which could serve the purpose of my inquiry and prepare me to meet others. With Nithya, the plan was to spend whatever time she wanted to, share our stories and eat together on that hot summer day in 2017.

Noon was still an hour away when she got into my car. Our connection was quick, the ground having been laid in the phone conversation a few days ago. She was one of them who had responded to my request for participants via social networks. There was no further ado and now we both held the bull by the horns, ready to delve into painful, hitherto hidden stories of our lives.

Like Borg (2007:26), I believe crucially important knowledge comes from individuals with lived experience of mental health problems. Therefore, meeting with peers matters, even though and contrary to expectation, it was not straightforward notwithstanding (my) considerable lived experience. As I delve into those struggles ahead, my overriding focus remains centring peers' testimonies.

Two ideas inform the choice of design and its execution here: *recovery* and *epistemic viability*.[1] At the outset, I knew recovery was possible, for

---

1 In Chapter 2, I have referred to this as epistemic privilege and epistemic marginalization as two sides of the process of epistemic injustice, to denote one view appears to be more viable and one repeatedly undermined.

      DOI: 10.4324/9781003248804-4

experience generated curiosity, to look for similar others. Colin Hay (in Hiruy, 2014:6) notes that our ontological position and underpinning assumptions about what is knowledge influence our epistemology – what and how we think we can know – and in turn, our epistemological position influences our methodology and methods. I had little doubt recovery occurs, an ontological departure from the perspective "mental illness" is lifelong. I was not merely looking for recovery but further evidence. Illness and recovery are subjective evaluations which may/not be approved by "experts". It is the knowledge of people, or what they themselves evaluate as source(s) of their distress that needs acknowledgement. To reach its bottom was my first goal, and among all options I chose to understand experience via the narrative.

Working through narrative

"Mental illness" has often been represented by stakeholders other than "patients",[2] or when "patients" speak they are but one among several social representations. While professional representations are made by psy-professionals, government bureaucrats, legal professionals, caregivers, academics, non-profits, journalists and the media, these perspectives often gloss over individual subjectivities, being easy to cast aside for lacking credibility.

I prioritize peer voices beyond all prevailing prejudice, and these are what I represent over others. Referring to the seminal contribution of Gayatri Spivak in the context of groups who are silenced, Dotson (2011:236) confirms that a method of executing epistemic violence is to damage a given group's ability to speak and be heard. Due to Spivak and other philosophers, the reality that members of oppressed groups can be silenced by virtue of group membership is widely recognized (ibid.).

Listening to a story from the bearer of the experience is paramount and marks a peer's efforts to respond to the silenced. Hence, I settled for working with narratives, in whatever manner peers chose to share, albeit in a semi-structured format. Hyden (1997:49) concurs one of our most powerful forms for expressing suffering is the narrative. Such inquiry offers a scope for collaboration between researcher and participants, over time, in a place or series of places, and in social interaction with milieus (Clandinin & Connelly, 2000:20). For a researcher, the choice of narrative as a method for evoking stories seems natural, non-intimidating. Narrative inquiry studies experience which researchers utilize to give voice to suppressed minorities or the otherwise demeaned, facilitating greater social understanding

2 My current focus is research testimonies, though there is considerable representation of lived experience as memoirs, biographies, autobiographies, etc., from all parts of the world.

suggest Clandinin and Connelly (Gergen and Gergen, 2011:377). Though people given a "psychosis" diagnosis are not seen "suppressed" in a traditional sense, but due to identity prejudice (Fricker, 2007), their representations and knowledge are undermined, marginalized, considered unreliable.

Following a narrative sensibility, this chapter is also one such. It captures the story of this book having ethical, relational and methodological sides. It tells the reader how I met the peers whose stories appear here, acquired the means to understand their stories beyond diagnostic labels via the epistemic structure you encountered earlier, how I arrived at these ideas and related issues.

My idea to unravel barriers begins from the idea that talking to others who deal with them may bring clarity. I had little idea where/all they could lie. My first goal was to meet people, a process which was complex for its own reasons as you have read, and only later to see what law had to say about recovery. Primarily, the endeavour was to learn with peers, either from them directly or through the dialogues that occurred between us, for dialogues are often generative. Peer narratives shed light on the micro-aspects of recovery, while legal and human sciences' literatures constitute macro-aspects illuminating structural barriers for recovery. The interaction between the micro- and macro-variables constitutes the kernel of this book, necessitating this interdisciplinary investigation. I examine legal, medical and social provisions for recovery and consequently achieve two goals, responding to two constituencies.

A study of existing recovery options clarifies the scope law creates to help individual recovery, which it may by offering non-psychiatric options for recovery, non/insistence on drug compliance or creating different infrastructure for recovery. Empirical research gathers evidence and understandings from "patient" and caregiver perspectives about what does/not support recovery in the macro-environment. This constitutes the larger framework wherein I examine how recovery is conceptualized in India's mental health legislations and its compliance with the CRPD.

The design

My exploration of recovery draws on three research programs (Patti Lather, 1986:258). The first is collaborative[3] inquiry from social construction. The second is emancipatory research enriched by critical pedagogy, disability studies and emancipatory-survivor research. The third component, also part of my positionality (Chap.1), is what is construed the "insider-outsider" space. Earlier in research, the status of the researcher was either an insider

---

3 From the beginning this collaboration was not planned beyond the data collection stage due to the geographically distributed nature of peers in this book. They are not involved in narrative analysis.

or an outsider. "Exploring the insider-outsider status in terms of position-ality ... can be a time to discover tools for understanding the dynamics of researching within and across a researcher's own social group or culture" (Crean, 2018:para.3). Crean notes further it specifically becomes a research tool for minority scholars within academia to use "insider-outsider" sta-tus to reconnect with their community and group of origin and further develop alternative forms of knowledge and ways of knowing and under-standing the social world. When researchers were either insiders or outsid-ers of the populations they researched, both positions had dis/advantages. Researchers (Merriam et al. 2001:405) view these positions as complex, with boundaries not clearly delineated or a continuously reshaped dilemma (Rose, 2019). My experience of having been *inside* the mental health system makes me an insider of both "psychosis" and its "treatment". Currently, I am neither part of the mental health system as "patient"[4] nor part of any peer's life whose story appears here I am the *outsider.*

Peer-research signifies research led or controlled by those who have similar experiences of what they research. Emancipatory researchers are not "outsiders" who study purely from academic or scholarly curiosity. We bring insights, politics and ken to cultural phenomena, attempting to broaden understandings by looking beyond the personal into sociological contexts where they originate. We also look at the impact of the sociologi-cal on the individual in a bi-directional flow, for the insider role is precisely that: being and experiencing what the peer experiences now or in the past. We bring scope for reciprocal exchange, for few inquire into a researcher's personal story in other research designs.

When non-disabled researchers study others, their perspectives fall in two broad categories: positivist (normative) and interpretive. Until recently, the socio/medical model of disability has been dominated by interpreta-tive studies of the experience of "illness", which focus on individual cop-ing mechanisms, including management of "stigma", and other "perceived threats to self and identity" says Bury (in Barnes and Mercer, 1997:3). At times, researchers have ignored how biological and social factors are sources of social disadvantages experienced by disabled people. Research-ers of all methodological persuasions have consistently misunderstood and distorted both the phenomenon of disability and the experiences of the disabled people (Oliver, 1992:101–102).

Meeting peers and their families

I slid my small car towards the left curb at the metro station. We were both tired yet, speaking for myself, touched by the other's story. It was past six

---

4 Though I do offer peer services.

in the evening and the preceding seven hours had gone in a mix of listening, writing, discussion, sharing, eating, drinking summer sherbets or tea while intermittently recording. I was tired, not having had the afternoon rest one is accustomed to. At two decades my younger Nithya betrayed little sign of similar fatigue, but there was no way to tell. I was relieved we would soon part, for the data she had shared was considerable. It needed time to get my head around it. I had taken written permission, from her and other peers in this book, for writing, recording and representing their narratives. In exchange, I offered my own. While the former is an ethical commitment of qualitative research, the latter stems from emancipatory research.

In the midst of writing as she spoke, I figured an attentive listening was better than desperate attempts to scribble along, trying to catch fleeting words or experiences. Not being a fan of multitasking, I found myself losing out words or phrases as she recalled from memory; naturally enough someone narrating their life talks in a flow, its speed may be difficult to capture in writing. Simultaneously posing questions and writing is stressful. I laid my pen, simply listened and asked questions, letting recording take care of memory lapses if/when they would occur. Then onward, this remained the format for all interactions.

***

Two months later

I rang the doorbell and was ushered in. Nithya and her father welcomed me, the summer now her humid monsoonal version. The scorching heat felt stifling, but the apartment was cool. Her parents were waiting expectantly; it would not have been possible otherwise. They remained guarded the entire time I stayed. So much so her father kept telling me to come inside to sit in one of the inner rooms, lest neighbours heard. I assured him nobody saw me come and why would anyone want to put their ears to the walls, snooping on their life? This was unusual to comprehend, for the stresses of every life are unique, somewhat unimaginable for an outsider you do not share context with.

Over the next few hours, we went over another investigation of our respective narratives. Before myself, I let them have the prerogative, as part of my ethical posture, to ask any number of questions or discuss at length whatever I knew about recovery including about my personal one. Thereafter, they poured their anxieties, the challenges they faced, or how they tried overcoming them, in what ways they were trying to help their daughter. While we communicated, Nithya sat through our deliberations and happily chipped in wherever she felt necessary, later contributing to the meal we shared.

Interestingly, while she did not want anyone to be present when we had met she would not leave her parents alone to talk! Even more interestingly, in future wherever I spoke with any parents who are caregivers, their "children"[5] usually wanted to be present somewhere in the vicinity while not wanting parental presence when we spoke between us. I too was keen to hear peers' unmediated testimonies, without passing them through filters of parental presences or worldviews. So I never questioned this choice. The goal was to understand individual by individual their versions of what had led them to seek psychiatric intervention, who played what role in the past or present, how they had been supported, or not, or continued supporting their loved one/s as "patients".

Relational aspects of research

MR. MEHTA: *"So madam what did you do to recover?"*
ME: *"There were many things that brought about the change Mr. Mehta. If you would like to know I have written at least a few articles about them, you are welcome to read them. They were mostly academic and musical activities. I do not know what to tell you here, or in what way my story can help you".*

I had little clarity whether musical or academic pursuits led to my recovery for none was a university-based learning associated with career goals. There were more variables I had no clarity about that supported recovery. In writing autoethnographic narratives while I had captured certain aspects of my recovery, it was not a socio-cultural abstraction yet, to be offered as template for other recoveries. For that, patterns across narratives would have to become clearer; the quest I was undertaking.

I sat on the *diwan* in their living room, while Mr. Mehta sat on a chair at a little distance. Their house was a long way from home, the only occasion I interviewed both a peer and their caregiver on the same day. I had little money to spend on taxi fare, and the distance seemed considerable. Although there were plans to meet others in this area, this occasion decided it for me. Another taxi ride to meet anyone in the National Capital Region of Delhi was ruled out, instead I chose to interview on phone.

Hetal, Mr. Mehta's daughter, had emailed me several months earlier inquiring whether I could counsel her mother. I requested them to come to my home-office from where I operate my counselling practice. Both mother and daughter had a schizophrenia diagnosis, yet the daughter was seeking help for the mother, not herself. Months passed by they never came, partially perhaps, due to distance. When I feel short of contributors to this study, I thought of everyone who had ever approached me for counselling,

---

5 The youngest person at the time I gathered their stories was 22 and the oldest 60. While nobody was a "child" in a developmental sense, "children" refers to adults who live with their parents as caregivers, an existing social norm in India.

and never made it. This family was one among them. I wrote to the daughter requesting them to contribute to this study. She is one of two individuals in this book with a family history of "psychosis".

Mr. Mehta appeared as the caregiver of both, though his wife was also mentioned in the consent form as a caregiver to their daughter. When we met, I understood the daughter was in a calmer frame than her mother; the latter restless, uneasy. She kept searching my face from a distance and glided around quietly, without sitting down for any of our dialogues. Neither among them smiled at me. I don't know if it was because I had declined their request to counsel the mother when I visited them, for it was ethically untenable. Possibly, it made me appear only a nuisance then – sifting through their stories. Though I have met many parents and caregivers meeting Mr. Mehta was somewhat unique. Here was a father insisting to know my recovery story, asking the same question in different ways. I had nothing new to add, for I hardly understood recovery then the manner I do now. He seemed to work like a detective, as though trying to extract something hidden which sufficient interrogation would make me divulge. He could not understand my absolute lack, or *epistemic ignorance* for while the story of my recovery lay in my head, it was neither fully documented nor generalizable. It wasn't as if I was holding back something; my knowledge itself was insufficient.

He persisted, *"there is something you would have done that you could recover. What exactly is it? I mean how is it that you could recover, whereas doctors never say anyone can"*.

He was right. I too had not heard from any psychiatrist someone can recover, nobody is expected to. My psychiatrist, whenever I consulted him insisted I still needed medication "just a little longer". He repeated so for years no matter after how long we met. How much I waited for him to hint that I could stop, but it never happened, at least not from his end.

> *I think everyone needs to be engaged in some form of rehabilitation. That is what I too did, it helped me recover. But yes I also switched over to homeopathy. It is all in the public domain.*
>
> I explained again

At least whatever I knew about my recovery was out in the open, there was not an extra ounce hidden.

> *That is fine Madam; we also tried many other paths. I took them to Balaji[6] temple, and they do many things. But there are still some issues lingering. I am trying to see what more can be done.*

---

6 Further details in Chapter 4.

He was not buying the idea that homeopathy was the solution, nor I could vouch for it but suggest only as an option.

He tried returning to the question as we talked. I felt strangely cornered as though accused of denying information. In general, he was not willing to live with the uncertainty of "not knowing", a stance social construction prepares someone for (Anderson, 1997:64). His world appeared one of certainties and "fixities"; when someone did not supply the necessary material for such "fixing", perhaps the person need not be further engaged with.[7] Thinking about it, later I felt suspect, my claim to research as though an "extraction" – "growing" at their expense, "robbing" them of their stories, not offering something commensurate. I understood his concern as a caregiver to both his wife and daughter, yet I could not then convey my own ignorance, being equally unaware!

I came away from this meeting tired from the distance, the heat and crestfallen with the interaction, to be greeted by my canine family – all four eagerly barking, jumping on me. Meeting Mr. Mehta and his family offered confirmation why some people[8] want to engage with us – "ex-patients". They feel we carry some lock to unlock a hidden vault of information about recovery which can be extricated if they persist long enough. It is not a peer relationship or connection they seek, but to utilize a relational possibility in an instrumental sense: to serve their purpose, "elicit" information.

These interactions with research contributors constitute the social relations of research production, which Oliver (1992) builds an argument to examine closely as they provide a structure within which research is undertaken. Social relations are built on a firm distinction between the researcher and the researched, with an underlying belief it is the researchers who have specialist knowledge and skills (Oliver, 1992:102). Building a historical schema of research production Oliver distinguishes three stages of the evolution of research, viz., the positivist, interpretive and the emancipatory stage.

Recognizing this distinction, this book is an emancipatory effort to steer clear of those distortions which "professional" researchers' gaze creates. I attempt to centralize the voice of the "mentally ill", to wrest free of psychiatric interpretation of our suffering and reclaim our right to speak for ourselves in a language that is not distorted, interpreted or transformed into another professional language. The agenda of my work is to restore our own epistemic existence (Liegghio, 2013:127). The importance of emancipatory research paradigm lies in how it attempts to challenge existing power relations, as also the demystification of the ideological structures

---

7 This is exactly what he did when I tried to tell him later about my findings, he never took my call!

8 I routinely encounter clients in my counselling practice who often come with a similar attitude.

within which these power relations are located (Oliver, 1992:110). He further invites attention emancipatory disability research ought to attempt a change in the social relations of research production. Such an enterprise can be about the self-understanding of researchers as well as researched and it need not be separated from wider processes of education and politics (Oliver, 1992:112). Time and again, I have endeavoured to offer a level playing field to peers, not manipulate extracting narratives in a one-sided manner.

Gollop (in Oliver, 1992:111) flags three key fundamentals on which an emancipatory research paradigm must be based: *reciprocity, gain and empowerment*. It would be presumptuous to claim I have succeeded in meeting these goals with all peers. But envisioning these goals has ensured a connection with both mine and others' subjectivities. While I offered a reciprocal exchange, and gained further understanding from peer narratives, I regret I cannot claim the same for them, especially those who chose to sever our links in the years after our interactions.

Notwithstanding differences, some peers remain connected until today, while others are not even remotely connected. Mr. Mehta and his family are among the latter. Even though I tried sharing whatever I learnt, while it occurred my intention was misunderstood. My deliberation was *not* to make the venture an alienating experience for peers, a practice I maintain. As narratives were collected over the internet, it facilitated on-going interaction, feedback and exchange. It may have been different had my field and fieldwork not been so seamlessly interwoven.

Challenges of meeting peers

Gathering narratives was far from co-sharing with peers I had initially imagined. While narrative seemed an easy choice, executing it was not. Challenges appeared from unexpected quarters, especially those I thought simple issues like gaining access to peers or finding enough number of narratives for this work. I was unprepared to encounter silences in response to my request for recruiting contributors, thinking I knew enough people everywhere who may want to talk with me. Months of sending emails, messages, phone calls and public requests did not yield the number of participants I had planned for. I was forced to think of an alternate path: inviting people known to me. People who have a "psychosis" diagnosis and treatment are not so widely distributed or publicly visible that I had numerous options. I finally approached many from different kinds of networks, created over years of research – well before my current study. As I illustrated above, some were prospective clients, who never forged a counselling relationship.

I encountered widespread reluctance among "patients" and their families to participate in this study. Being unprepared for "silence" from people known to me, some responses took me by surprise, especially those who had been promising from the beginning they would participate. In fact, it unnerved me considerably. Scott and Geddes (2016:124) caution about an initially overambitious and simplistic view of our peer/community "insider" status. At least here was one area I presumed where it was certain to find cooperation, for it was an issue close to us all. Peer-hood I thought offered a scope to create affinity, trust and connection and as Faulkner (2004:3) suggests for survivor research, empowerment, clarity and transparency. To some extent, subsequent interactions confirmed this, but silences pushed me towards creating multimodal pathways for recruiting peers.

Researchers bring their own attitudes to the research process and clarifying it helps one remain transparent. Getting someone to tell you their life story is, under any circumstances, a delicate process (Mazza, 2016:73). Memory is reconstructed, not merely recalled.

> [H]ow can a contributor as an expert on his or her everyday life provide us with access to the domain of his or her original experience? Simply and only by describing his or her experiences to us as closely and faithfully as possible to the ways in which they were originally experienced. In other words, rather than asking a person to explain his or her experiences *to* us, we are asking him or her to share his or her experiences with us: to tell us stories about his or her life as he or she lived it.
>
> (Davidson, 2003:63)

In inviting peers, I have often negotiated this delicate balance of what to ask, or not. At times the medium of our communication, especially when phone, proved a challenge. Yet all research is shaped by the subjective experiences of researcher's choices, mine no exception. Inviting people into dialogues opens room for a respectful engagement. I have tried it in all earnest.

Relationship with peers

In peer research, shared experiences become cornerstones which enable access to research contributors. In a peculiar way, a majority of peer meetings began with them interviewing me first. As Faulkner (2004) recommends, I have maintained transparency at all levels – about the nature of my research, my life and on-going connections. In some or another way, I try remaining connected to all my research contributors, not entirely successfully. Like feminist scholars Duncombe and Jessop (2002), I wonder whether career goals of researchers can make them "feign" rapport and friendship in trying to evoke narratives for their studies. They draw diverse examples from their researches in which their professional goals and needs made them to "fake" friendships, with their research participants. This in turn raises ethical dilemmas and questions which they explore elaborately. Thompson

(2002:99) also wonders about a potentially "pseudo-intimate" nature of research. He flags at least three consent difficulties which are "expectations of friendship", "participants" sharing "too much" and "voluntariness".

Peer researchers[9] may have a different set of values and attitudes than other researchers.[10] My understanding of peers' suffering mirrors my own; it is not just an intellectual or professional quest. The personal is a vivid part of memory and a point of reference for gaining further insights to others' struggles. Even though a majority of peers in this book do not have the length of experience of "psychosis" I have, it doesn't make me question the nature of their suffering or masquerade concern or friendship. My response has been of offering accounts of my struggles or the manner I have dealt with obstacles in all earnest. While there is no doubt that it is a valid concern how researchers may "fake" connection for their career goals, but peer research has taken me back to those known to me for considerable amounts of time. Instead of faking concern, this book is built on longstanding relationships in a number of cases.

Power dynamics

There are concerns about asymmetrical power relationship between researchers and participants in research interviews, and potential oppressive use of interview-produced knowledge (Kvale, 2006:483). Instruments of power may also be a manipulative dialogue, and an act in which the researcher holds a monopoly over interpretation (ibid: 485). I mention these partially in recognition of their meaningfulness and partly to respond.

I have said earlier my interactions have not been one-sided questioning, but a reciprocal exchange. Neither can feign suffering which "psychosis" conjures for people. Equally so not many have met a peer who is a researcher, or an "ex-patient". Most connections forged or reinforced for this work did not get over, they continue.

Analysing narratives

My approach to analysis lies in unraveling the socially constructed outcomes of language using insights from Critical Discourse Analysis (CDA). Language and its usage are acts of social construction; they create and perpetuate power structures. Hodge and Kress (in Machin and Mayr, 2012:2–3) argue "language is a form of social practice ... intertwined with how we act and how we maintain and regulate our societies ... Through language,

---

9 This is also my experience as a research informant in another survivor-controlled research.

10 I confirm this both as researcher and peer having contributed in other research done by peers.

certain kinds of practices, ideas, values and identities are promoted and naturalized"; others are marginalized.

Language holds significance for diverse scholars and researchers, especially since the most recent philosophical revolution, in Linguistic Philosophy. Rorty (1992:3) notes that philosophical problems are problems which may be solved (or dissolved) either by reforming language or by understanding more about the language we presently use. This view is considered by many of its proponents to be *the most important philosophical discovery of our time*, and, indeed, of the ages. I cannot but confirm the same.

Whether psychiatric diagnoses are actual medical conditions or linguistically arrived categories creates a need for a critical examination of language at an ethical and philosophical level. Therefore critical perspectives appeal to me. Social constructionism also centralizes language and proposes that mutually agreed upon ideas or discourse among members of a group create categories or establish certain claims to knowledge. The idea that "mental illness" is a social construction dressed in the language of medical "expertise" in noteworthy.

> Informed by a constructionist sensitivity, we are challenged to step out of the realities we have created, and to ask significant questions – what are the repercussions of these ways of talking, who gains, who is hurt, who is silenced, what traditions are sustained, which are under-mined, and how do I judge the future we are creating? Such questioning does not proceed effortlessly – with methods tried and true. It is not easy in part because we live these discourses.
> (Gergen, 1999:62)

However, while language is central to many philosophical and research traditions, I am drawn to the interaction between language, discourse and social power, or how they are streams falling into the same river.

Critical discourse analysis (CDA)

CDA is a form of *critical* social analysis (Fairclough, 2018:13). Critical social analysis shows how forms of social life can damage people unnecessarily, but also how they can be changed. Most kinds of CDA will ask questions about the way specific discourse structures are deployed in the reproduction of social dominance (van Djik, 2001:353–354). The dominance I focus on is psychiatry's: through prevalent discourse, legal and penal institutions at its disposal or its ability to formulate policies to further its goals and purposes. What indeed are its ways to naturalize its discourse? "All social practices are ... the means by which existing social relations are reproduced or contested and different interests are served.

It is the questions pertaining to interests that relate discourse to relations of power" (Janks, 1997: 329).

In Chapter 2, I discussed the nature of psychiatric discourse and how it becomes hegemonic. In recent times, discourse has come to be used in place of ideology (Holborow, 2007:52). She questions Foucauldian emphasis on discursive regimes, which downplays the social and economic foundations of power. I agree language being an instrument of power also operates in an ideological milieu whose basis is determined by capital. Effectively, language becomes an instrument of maintaining, reinforcing and extending the goal of any ideology.

> Because ideology crystallizes in language, ideology can appear as if frozen in language. Repeated from the lofty heights of the media and positions of power, these ideological representations can acquire the status of natural truths and common sense. This was the significant insight that Gramsci made when he identified that this uncritical acceptance was part of how ruling ideas won consent, or hegemony.
>
> (Holborow, 2007:53)

van Djik (2007:14–15) agrees that ideologies form the basic social representations of the beliefs shared by a group and precisely function as the framework which defines the overall coherence of these beliefs. Thus, ideologies allow new social opinions to be easily inferred, acquired and distributed in a group when the group and its members are confronted with new events and situations. Inasmuch as we operate in a neo-liberal world, which is dominated by a capitalist ideology, we are socialized into believing about ourselves and our worlds by the dominant class, the capitalist, and every linguistic choice is made to favour the interests of the same. Fairclough (1989:3) reminds us ideology is pervasively present in language. This ought to mean the ideological nature of language should be one of the major themes of modern social science. He repeatedly draws attention to how language becomes an instrument of power or how language contributes to the domination of some people by others. He offers a schema how this dominance is established via text and then discursively disseminated.

Michael Hardt and Tony Negri (in Holborow, 2007:55) believe language itself maintains social hierarchies – within and across communities "as a relationship between power and knowledge". The idea of "mental illness" pathology succeeds as a social representation and gains acceptance due to the social power of the professional, including resources to make herself heard. It is enacted because the social representation of the professionals is accorded greater validity and acceptability, vis-à-vis self-representations by "patients". Language does not offer an equalizing scope for both groups.

I tease out *this* inequality via CDA. My interest lies in examining how this inequality is enacted.

I utilize CDA to make sense of peer narratives and their experiences negotiating psychiatric power.

> This means that although our experiences are all *qualitatively* distinct, they are always still open to being "worded" in countless different ways – with each "wording" opening up not only different possible ways of acting in the future, but also of bringing to light *relations* and *connections* with other experiences not previous recognized.
>
> (Shotter, 2016:6)

I specifically focus on psychiatric labelling, by examining the discursive landscape it impacts in day-to-day lives of people.

van Dijk (2015:467) summarizes the tenets of CDA as having the following features

- It focuses primarily on *social problems* and *political issues* rather than the mere study of discourse structures outside their social and political contexts.
- This critical analysis of social problems is usually *multidisciplinary*.
- Rather than merely *describe* discourse structures, it tries to *explain* them in terms of properties of social interaction and especially social structure.
- More specifically, CDA focuses on the ways discourse structures enact, confirm, legitimate, reproduce or challenge relations of *power abuse* (*dominance*) in society.

Considering the above features, it may be clear CDA is not confined to a particular method of analysis. Fairclough (2003:6) confirms CDA can draw upon a wide range of approaches to analysing text. I look into different contexts of people's lives and see what options they have and how they choose what they do, considering their bargaining power.

To embark upon the analytical task, I follow Janks' (1997:329) recommendation of Fairclough's approach to CDA. She commends it as useful for it offers multiple points of analytic entry. In this model, there are three interrelated processes of analysis which are tied to three interrelated dimensions of discourse, viz., (1) the object of analysis, (2) the process of producing and receiving the object and (3) the sociohistorical conditions that govern these processes. Since I work with text elicited from interviews, the object of analysis resides in those texts or narratives.

I illustrate this approach with an example.

ME: *"So if you have anxiety is there anybody you can talk to?"*
VINDHYA: *"Anxiety, ma'am … I--I lose the relationships ma'am when I am (having) anxiety and people, they don't come back to me after … after I … (have) spoken something in when I am--I am (experiencing) anxiety".*

I asked Vindhya whether there is someone she can communicate to alleviate her anxiety, especially in emergencies. She appears reluctant to reach out to others even in her vicinity. Perhaps, the reluctance has a past connection, for whoever she reached out to seeking help distanced themselves. In requesting for help, she got further isolated and her relationships suffered. So she is left alone to deal with anxiety; the individual grappling with "schizophrenia" rendered helpless, instead of supported by her social world.

This is the manner of my analysis using CDA, applying it to the chosen text. As Janks (1997) proposes, citing Fairclough, there are multiple dimensions of analysis: the description, interpretation and explanation. Vindhya's words give testimony of her lack of social support in precisely those moments when she requires it most. Lacking it, she has chosen to not seek it, instead remain quiet and go through her anxieties alone! This statement is textually analysed and then interpreted in the context of the speaker and a social analysis is offered. From the latter, I derive why someone with a "schizophrenia" diagnosis may appear reluctant to seek help. This is my approach to analysis.

II

MAPS OF RECOVERY

> Perhaps the greatest tragedy of modern man is his domination by the force of these myths and his manipulation by organized advertising, ideological or otherwise... Ordinary men do not perceive the tasks of the time; the latter are interpreted by an "elite" and presented in the form of recipes, of prescriptions. And when men try to save themselves by following the prescriptions, they drown in leveling anonymity, without hope and without faith, domesticated and adjusted.
>
> Freire (1974:5)

The myth of mental illness (Szasz: 2010) is so well entrenched it is presumed "truth". The manner this truth is routinized is not a simple diffusion of *scientific ideas* based on objective truths but professional groups working for expansion of their agenda, medicalizing ordinary experiences of living as mental health issues. When "experts" offer overarching "science based" explanations for people's suffering, the latter are left with little choices but to accept their prescriptions and recommendations. Hence, few think of going beyond "expert" opinions; never finding the courage to exit the "paternal" gaze of the professional.

The professional is the gatekeeper who guards the lay person and assures her to stay within the institution where her *interests are best protected*. But for recovery it is precisely this gatekeeper one has to get past, which a majority never does. In this mythic template people once inside the mental health system stay confined without ever developing the capacity to question experts. Yet there are some who can.

Recovery occurs in this minuscule number given a "psychosis" diagnosis, the rest simply play the patient role. There are barriers which do not let a majority recover while some do. Where do these barriers exist? Are they individual, interpersonal or systemic barriers? Are such barriers universal or are they more individualistic? What is the way to resolve this?

DOI: 10.4324/9781003248804-5

Two kinds of empirical investigation throw light on the nature of barriers to recovery. The first is a human sciences inquiry of "patient" and caregiver narratives. People who recover have other facilitators, requiring further probe into their life trajectories. The second is a doctrinal inquiry from an interdisciplinary perspective examining the institutional framework, access to services mandated by Indian law and policy and nature of services available to the average citizen when they require mental health support.

The goal of this section is to apprise the reader that barriers to recovery exist in diverse forms, varying from single to multiple, and intersectional barriers. While the goal is not to specify what barrier impacts which individual, by the analyses that follow a spectrum of barriers are teased out. In Chapter 4, they are identified as the micro barriers embedded in relational networks, and in Chapter 6, their trail is traced to the legal-policy frameworks, whereupon they are classified macro barriers. In Chapter 5, those narratives where peers successfully recover are scrutinized for how they managed, whereas others remain bound in psychiatric webs.

4

"BENIGN" ARM OF PSYCHIATRY AND BIRTH OF THE PSYCHIATRIC SUBJECT

The voice of the ill person is made possible by modernist medicine, but it cannot be contained within modernist assumptions, particularly those about medical professional dominance and the narrative surrender this dominance requires. A divide has been crossed into new territory, the post-modern, and we know this crossing by the new voices[1] that are heard.

(Frank, 1997:18)

"I was agitated ... at times feel suffocated at home. I would go out and walk a lot, be by myself. That used to be a relief, otherwise I would be very suffocated ... And I also felt a change in the behavior of people. I don't know if it was a change in my thinking or their behavior was as such. Or ... it was becoming too much for me to handle. Then I just went to Bombay (to escape my family for a while). Upon my return my dad took me to a physician and he said take her to a psychiatrist."[2] – Bhavna.

This narration by a peer captures her pathway of referral and may appear a simple referral by a general physician to a specialist. Her words, in fact, veil a complex, surreptitious process at work: transforming a person to a "patient", from a free citizen to someone who would soon be facing silent, unspoken panopticonic[3] surveillance from numerous others around, from

---

1 "New voices" refers to peer testimonies which were not credible until they got represented by another peer. Not only this but all Mad Studies scholarship does similarly.
2 Regular italics indicate peer and caregiver testimonies and bold italics when they quote someone.
3 This is a system of the Panopticon, an architectural edifice where the warden in a central tower can monitor the prisoners in their cells without the prisoners seeing their warden (Walia, 2021).

DOI: 10.4324/9781003248804-6

a person until recently defining her selfhood to one who would learn to review herself through the objectified knowledge of psychiatry. The person is not only becoming a patient, but also a subject.

Subject and subjectivation

There is a traditional understanding of self, defined by the great 19th-century deterministic models of Sigmund Freud, Karl Marx and Charles Darwin. These models initiated a rethinking of just how unique humans were as individuals by emphasizing how much we are shaped by biological and economic forces. The postmodern theory of the subject, however, depends on another revolution that in linguistics, especially the structuralist linguistics of the Swiss linguist Saussure (Ganim, 2005:225). Structuralist and poststructuralist theories have taken the system of language as a model and questioned whether an autonomous self can exist in any society. This theorization has significant implications for the present context wherein though the autonomous self may seem to exist, in reality it is does not.

> These theories have attempted to replace the terminology of the "self" with the terminology of the "subject". In so doing, we are made to confront the possibility that the coherent, autonomous, fully conscious self is an illusion. As with the notion of the subject in grammar, the subject is acted upon, even constituted, by other discourses. We are not the conscious centres[4] of awareness we think we are, but are sites upon which various forces – psychological, sociological, economic, and political – act and intersect.
>
> (ibid.)

A person seeking help is similarly acted upon by a set of ideas and discourse prevalent in society about how they can be helped. They too are willing to surrender their subjective truth(s) and accept the notion of "pathology". Nobody simply becomes a "patient" because an authoritative person said so: they tacitly agree being subjected to psychiatric treatments in the belief it will bring respite. As Ganim pointed above, the choice of seeking particular treatments occurs in a milieu where the self faces different points of view, each capable of defining suffering uniquely: from biology, to family issues, economic factors or other sources. One does not become a "patient"

---

4 Original spellings by author.

if they do not agree their suffering has roots beyond their comprehension. In this book, one peer rejects this biomedical, reductionist view. Therefore, his and his parental narratives provide important insights.

Yet one question is more pertinent: does one choose to become a psychiatric "subject", or do they choose "treatment"? This foundational issue leads to further questions. If one only knew they were about to surrender their autonomy in choosing a "treatment", and henceforth only an objective "truth" will prevail about them, would they still choose it? People are neither aware of this trade-off nor of their entry into a colonizing relationship (see Chapter 2). Time and again, individuals refer each other and themselves to psychiatric clinics with an attitude of trust and surrender, reposing it in their relationships with psychiatrists. Everyone hopes whatever their distress, it will be suitably addressed and healed. In their unquestioning submission, there is a belief which

> reflects that applied science is for a liberal not a mere set of instruments and methods ... but taken as *good* and *absolute*. There is no question that science can be anything but. It is taken as a given that since a man of science, a doctor in this case, is applying science in the "best interest" of his patient, his motives, ethical assumptions, means and goals could remain unquestioned, implicit, above board and honorable.
>
> (Burke, 1969:30)

To arrive at the idea of subjectivation, I interrogate the micro-politics of social power in the lives of distressed individuals, which enables this process. The focus here lies on "patient" and caregiver voices and their struggles for recovery. To accomplish it, barriers established by modernist medicine or their representation of "patients" as case histories alone is overcome. The postmodern divide is crossed when people's own stories are no longer told as secondary but have their own primary importance (Frank, 1997:7). Peer narratives in this book do not play a secondary role, as partial testimonies which are either inadmissible or need other ratifications. They are credible truths and command recognition on their own merit.

These narratives are stitched together to elaborate on the making of the psychiatric subject. By doing this, I explicate on the presence of certain dominances within the mental health matrix and unearth their link with recovery. While putting narratives through a discourse analytic process I elucidate who becomes voiceless when "patients" and professionals deliberate. I am curious because the manner in which truths are produced about disorder also sustain "normality" and dominant forms of morality (Fullagar, 2017). It establishes a certain lens (of pathology) to look at and govern certain kinds of people: here identified "mentally ill". Subjectification, also called *subjectivation* by Foucault, refers to the procedures by which the subject is led to observe herself, analyse herself, interpret herself and recognize herself as a domain of possible knowledge: "the way the subject experiences [her]self in a game of truth where [s]he relates to [her]self" (Stewart and Roy, 2014:1877). To put it another way once, the "patient" understands her suffering stems from "pathology" she is more at ease and now confident of its remedy since it has come under the care of the "expert". With this accomplished, what is made out to be *the truth* about "mental illness" becomes accepted as reality, including by the "patient" who is now under its remit.

A diagnosis is only a first step in a longer process which makes people dependent upon psychiatrists for taking decisions in most areas of their lives, which in India may include day-to-day issues of choosing a career, marriage, parenting and more. The primacy of their "patient" self becomes the salient point of people's self-constructions; every life decision they make is by keeping an eye on their actual or assumed vulnerability as "patient". Becoming a psychiatric "patient" is not a simple issue of healthcare alone for psychiatric "patients" become medico-legal subjects the moment a psychiatric diagnosis is received (Davar, 2012:123). Unbeknown to them, their status has changed to medico-legal subjects; they can be coerced into whatever "treatment" is adjudged "in their best interest". Most only know of the medical side of their transformed lives, not the legal recalibration of their social position(s). This chapter investigates such subject formation or subjectivation, elaborating upon the pre-existing variables that become conduit(s) in the same.

Though scholarship in the field of mental health is already looking beyond the social construction of mental health and illness, to engage with post-structuralist debates that emphasize how power works through discourse to shape knowledge and subjectivity (Fullager, 2017), in this chapter, two things are attempted. First, by recreating vignettes, I illustrate the socially constructed aspects of diagnostic labels. Second, I analyse discursive practices of subjectivation, which establish individual pathology. Sociolinguistics proposes the process of making someone a subject as being socially contingent: "how language contributes to the domination of some people by others" (Fairclough, 1996:1). Upon interweaving narratives and their analysis, my goal is shedding light on how socially situated discursive practices contribute to subjectivation of the individual.

In the opening quote, Bhavna reveals a matrix of relationships which lead her towards psychiatric intervention. The mere fact that a referral comes from a physician forecloses her options to seek alternatives; more so since the referral is not just made to her, which she could have discretionarily ignored, but her father. The choice of treatment options available is dependent on many variables, each contributing towards subjectivation uniquely. In her case, the routine referral offered as expertise to (a) a close relative, (b) by a medical doctor, (c) in response to visible or experienced distress which may be a response

(d) or due to behavior of others and (e) the presence of a friend in Bombay are all factors, which in a fine capillary like manner, produce a synthesis where it is unanimously agreed her "abnormal" behavior needs "handling".

Narrative through a lens of subjectivation

Three themes are chosen here from peer narratives to scrutinize closely: (a) the role played by family, (b) adherence to psychiatric regimen and (c) rehabilitation efforts. The meta-commentary of this chapter comes from the idea of "subjecthood": people become subjects of something/someone. There were two ways Foucault differentiated between ideas of "subject to" and "making subject" (see Chapter 2). The latter is the focus here: how people *are made* subjects of psychiatry, for the purpose of *governing* them in a particular manner and how a particular form of objectified knowledge is imposed upon them – as governmental rationality.

Since becoming a psychiatric "patient" is not akin to becoming a patient of any other medical specialty,[5] in what manner are questions of subjects, subjectivity and subjectivation set in motion once someone receives a "mental illness" diagnosis? Is there awareness among "patients" about entering into subjecthood where their own subjectivity will soon be subsumed into a pre-existing category, edging out their unique self? Thereafter, in all likelihood, they will become subjects in the same manner the colonized become subjects of their colonial masters!

There is also a relational matrix within which subjectivation is accomplished. In each narrative someone apart from the distressed individual seeks psychiatric intervention for her. This person is trusted or (usually) related. Therefore, no doubts are raised about their beliefs, knowledge or ability to discern in the matter because they too are acting in the "best interest" of their loved one. Their recommendations become non-negotiable if the referral comes from a doctor, as Bhavna says above. Rebughini (2015:1) draws attention to considerations on subject, subjectivity and subjectivation as relational issues. She quotes Maeve Cooke who emphasizes the topic of ethics as the core element of subjectivity. "We must not conceptualize this capacity as a transcendent moral quality, but as a political and practical issue, related to the positions, the experiences, the expectations and the imagination of single subjects".

In psychiatric context, the ethics of treatment would ordinarily require potential "patients" at the outset be informed about their "illness", its prognosis, supplied the information that no immediate "cure" is being offered and the length of time for the "treatment" even if interminable. In day-to-day

---

5 A psychiatric diagnosis is mostly based on a reductionist observation by the psychiatrist and cannot be determined by any objective tests and measures making diagnosis a subjective evaluation, highly arbitrary and not a confirmed reality. This has been problematized by many researchers, (e.g., Cohen, 1993, Boyle, 2007, Sweet and Decoteau, 2017).

psychiatric practice, this does not happen. Psychiatrists have no trajectory or a plan for a "patient" to follow; it is mostly an unending "treatment". Their visible authority makes it impermissible for patient to question further. In fact, they insist it is a permanent condition, with brief phases of remission.

In front of my parents he changes his attitude and become friendly, supportive, even shaking hands. Doctor has not been listening despite it not working for me. But the problem is that with no doctors the outcomes will be any different.

–Nithya

In terms of the relational matrices, considerable amount of writing exists about how psychiatry establishes "mental illness" pathology (see Chapter 2). From these narratives, a structure emerges which broadly maps subjectivation. The structure, I propose as a three stage schema, reveals how people come under the remit of psychiatry and whether it ultimately leads to a long-term, chronic dependence on medication, a life centred around "patienthood" or whether they recover and integrate back into society. The schema is:

Stage I – Entering the relationship (with psychiatry)
Stage II – Entrainment or adjustment
Stage III – Consolidating or exiting the relationship

The analysis that follows is a description of the stages of this schema as it appears in individual narratives. Towards the end of this chapter, I weave these strands together all over again to suggest how the stages appear in every narrative. Thereafter, depending upon (rehabilitation) options, people settle for one of two outcomes: recover completely or become chronic *subjects/*"patients".

Help seeking, struggles and confusions

People seek medical help all the time and in a majority of cases accept the medical verdict unquestioningly. These days many may explore the internet or seek a second opinion. When experiencing mental distress few understand what is happening initially, or what afflicts them or their loved one.

She was very disturbed ... too disturbed. We did not know what to do. We even went to Balaji Mehendipur[6] ... only such people who are disturbed come there. We thought it may get better in a few days, for this is what we had been told as well.

– Mr. Mehta

6 For further detail see Satija, D.C., Nathawat, S.S., Singh, D. and Sharma, A. (1982). A study of patients attending Mehandipur Balaji temple – Psychiatric and psychodynamic aspects. *Indian Journal of Psychiatry*, 24(4): 375–379.

The family is often as troubled as the person experiencing distress; everyone is confused and anxious to help their loved one to their best. In getting to the root of the problem, they try everything within the range of their imagination, information and resources. Hetal's family visited a temple renowned for offering succour for mental health issues. The said temple is located in the Dausa district in Rajasthan, known as the Balaji temple of Mehendipur.

Similarly Smita was deeply disturbed due to the sudden death of a close relative leaving her parents confused about what was happening.

SMITA: *"We were wondering, we were wondering you know that ... what exactly ... what was the reason this was happening to me? I think once I was having turbulence in my mind".*

ME: *"Can you recall those voices or do you still hear them?"*

SMITA: *"Oh yeah I can, it ... it was very troubling for it was like somebody was stomping in my chest. It was like somebody was trying to say something through my chest".*

Smita's father shared they had trouble establishing what the matter with his daughter was, a trouble he said all parents experience. In Chapter 1, I noted how within the macro environment created by psychiatric discourse supported by law that individual stories unfold. This leads to options: how does the choice of treatment arise? The process of who is choosing what, at which social strata, where and at what costs, for getting "cured" of what, is a complex one (Davar, 2015:7). If someone has alternatives, they may probably not meet a psychiatrist first of all. But if society ostracizes faith healing, *ayurveda* or homeopathy, people are not left with choices but to seek psychiatric help. So whether or not alternatives exist or are sought after is not just a matter of individual choice, it also enjoys a social sanction. This ultimately leads to what is agreed upon to be legal and therefore legitimate. What is available is not just a matter of the law, for it is through the various institutions that people operate within, and through selective transmission of certain ideas through the media that people come to know about what option is available.

Whereas in all other medical areas, a diagnosis may be confirmed by clinical/ physical symptoms and/ or a test, in case of "mental illness", it is the word of the doctor alone that counts. The diagnosis is largely based on observation and discussion with caregivers – the sufferer does not know what it is about her that is being discussed. Everyone simply hopes some relief would be found and they often willingly and unknowingly participate in their own subjectivation! But who refers or accompanies someone to a psychiatrist first?

My sibling took me to the emergency room in Stanford University.
                                                              – Rupali, 41

My family members ... took me to a doctor.

– Jitendra, 60

The omnipresent biomedical discourse is readily available for people to look at and assess their behavior or that of others in their vicinity. Often people do not encounter the discourse directly – someone known, and trusted, introduces them to it. No matter how someone encounters psychiatry, it appears an empathetic, knowledgeable problem-solver capable of resolving their mental or behavioural crises. It appears as the benign arm of psychiatry – kind, benevolent, appearing to understand suffering and offering hope to end it. All peers in my study were either referred by someone or makes a self-referral into a socially established, agreed upon solution they considered competent to ameliorate their distress.

I told my father that I need to see a psychiatrist. Since there was one close to my house, we thought why not go, refer and seek opinion?

– Sona, 30

My mathematics teacher in school wrote a letter to my mother asking her to take me to a psychiatrist.

– Vindhya, 44

The analysis of power in the context of psychiatry can only be accomplished by viewing the interconnected actions of widely distributed agents working convergently,[7] enabled by a set of ideas/knowledge which is socially well entrenched, paternalistic and patriarchal, yet encounters little resistance or doubt. Goffman (1961:127) refers to this as the circuit of agents – "that participate fatefully in his (the 'patient's') passage from civilian to patient status". Initiation into the world of psychiatry is done through family, friends, teachers, colleagues and others. It appears most people are "taken" to a psychiatrist; they often do not choose it, with certain exceptions like Sona. People do not act autonomously in choosing psychiatric "treatments", at least mostly. They are acted upon by trusted others. Rupali and Jitendra were escorted by members of their families, Vindhya referred by a teacher, a figure whose authority would not be questioned ordinarily. In each instance, it appears someone else, whose view on the matter prevails, acts on their behalf. The individual is unable to judge or take this decision. Their agency is overshadowed by another's "guidance" or "recommendation", while they themselves adopt a more passive posture.

The process of becoming a subject of psychiatry has been set in motion at this juncture. Ironically, in this matter, "[t]he user often does not have the

---

7 Also see Appendix B.

choice of not buying the (psychiatric) services ... the user does not choose the product or service to be purchased. It is recommended by a doctor, who is also the provider or seller of the services" (Priya and Ghodajkar, 2018:4). These relationships reveal underlying patterns in their respective power dynamics, with different outcomes in every narrative.

At the first stage, when people are unaware about their distress, the struggle is to look for an explanation. Upon meeting a psy-professional, an explanation starts to take shape. But two other things happen simultaneously. The first is the inaugural of a stigmatized identity, which becomes a personal (and at times a social) reality and the second is a mortification of the person, as "[s]hame becomes a central possibility, arising from the individual's perception of one of his own attributes as being a defiling thing to possess, and one he can readily see himself as not possessing" (Goffman, 1963:7). The manner in which a human being is made subject to control and dependence and the manner in which a human being is "tied" to a specific identity through a conscience or self-knowledge constitute two aspects of a single, dynamic process, whose central feature according to Foucault is power, notes Roberts (2005:34). This power is further consolidated in the hands of psychiatry due to a prevailing consensus of it being the expertise knowledgeable of human suffering of this nature. Everyone looks up to psychiatric experts as a source of direction how to deal with this mortifying affliction.

People encounter the discourse of psychiatry in their day-to-day lives in a number of ways. Harper (2013:80) notes that psychiatric diagnosis is regularly discussed in the media, becoming part of everyday culture and so moving beyond the disciplinary boundary of psychiatry. This brings us to another key social function of diagnosis: that it appears to provide a legitimization of distress and disturbing conduct. Journalists' reports and television and cinema dramas depicting mental disorders are important influences (Jorm, 2000, Pirkis et al., 2006, Beachum, 2010, Hanley, 2015, Das et al., 2017, Haider, 2018, Parkinson, 2018, Reynolds, 2018, Srivastava et al., 2018). The prevalence of such a widely disseminated discourse appeals to people who connect with the ideas it propagates, as it seems legitimate, backed by science. Lay people often lack the knowledge and critical perspectives necessary to question such uniform representation of people's distress, while researchers often challenge such views. Boyle (2007:290–291) problematizes the manner in which diagnostic labels are established based upon a certain set of assumptions, as diagnostic concepts are not based on the kinds of research data needed to justify them and calls it ethically problematic, as it often imposed upon those who resist it.

But encountering a socially prevalent discourse and meeting a psychiatrist are different things. The question is when they personally experience distress in what manner do people interact with the discourse? Is it ready acceptance, denial, rejection or willingness to "surrender" to the sudden realization that they are now crossing a new threshold into (mental) pa-tienthood? And how do they negotiate their relationships with omniscient "experts"? Does this new-found relationship remain static, changeable, negotiable, dominating, mutual or something else? Are people able to as-sert their independent views with psychiatrists and become partners in their healing? Or, do they unquestionably submit to the "science-backed" expert recommendations? Suffice to say the relationship is fraught with struggles.

ME: *"Did you ever ask him what he was medicating you for?"*
BHAVNA: *"No I didn't ask him".*
ME: *"Did he give you a diagnosis?"*
BHAVNA: *"No, he said it was for depression … gave me Risperdal … for depression. Much later I came to know it is for schizophrenia".*

Bhavna's words are reminder of an existing social inequality where people are distinguishable on an axis of social power based on claims to knowl-edge and its privilege. Diagnosis plays a special role giving the diagnosing professional a social status. It brings social power construed vastly superior to the knowledge and power of those they diagnose. "Diagnostic disclo-sure … promoted the profession of medicine by transforming the doctor into purveyor of truth, vesting him with therapeutic powers, differentiating him from other practitioners and distinguishing him from the lay person" (Jutel, 2017:4).

Here psychiatry "performs" diagnosis; in a sweep establishing its dom-inance over the individual who is made a subject in the performance. The "patient" is not treated as a human worthy of respect and deserving of knowledge about their mind, body and its "treatment", but an unworthy knower who needn't even be informed about what they come to be relieved of. This attitude of the treating professional reveals the dominant wisdom within psychiatry that users understand very little of their own problems (Cohen, 2008:2). "Patients" have to be dealt with, even by deception if need be, or else by cheating, lying, forcefully or misleading, whatever the case may require. Indian psychiatry has several unique dilemmas to deal with, covert medication being one. Psychiatrists debate among themselves about its ethical posturing (e.g., Kala, 2012, Sarin, 2012). Commenting on how the liberal mind attributes an ethical conduct to the scientific minded spe-cialist, Kenneth Burke (1969:30) says that for the liberal minded, applied science is

not a mere set of instruments and methods … it is a *good* and *absolute,* and is thus circuitously endowed with the philosophic function of *God* as the grounding of values. His thinking thus vacillates indeterminately between his overt claims for science as sheer method, as sheer coefficient of power, and his covert claims for science as a substance which, like God, would be an intrinsically *good* power.

In traditional societies like India, the status of *God* is indeed reserved for the medical specialist, projected on the doctor, for the doctor is said to be capable of bringing a god-like healing touch and relief from suffering.

Bhavna's narrative, at the start of this chapter, inaugurates the tone for the narrative demystification that follows. Here there may be a semblance of the doctor, "patient" and caregiver/s being in a dialogic exchange, yet power is surreptitiously skewed towards the professional. Therefore, Burke (1969:141) encourages one to ask "[j]ust how does the hierarchic principle work in this particular scheme of equality?". The power of the professional is reinforced by a social web of institutions, while "patients" and caregivers remain unaware of the larger structural aspects of their relationship with psychiatry. It is a belief in the ethics of science, they trust working in their favour, accepted uncritically. Consequently, their belief in doctors and treatments is akin to a religious belief. When the doctor gives a diagnosis, there is no resistance – partially because people do not understand its meaning, and partially due to the attitude of surrender and belief they bring to the relationship.

Descent into "psychosis": reconfiguring distress as diagnosis

To trace the emergence of acute distress in individual stories if we trace them to the social webs people are embedded in, they take a socially constructed dimension. What distress pushes people to seek psychiatric intervention? I asked my peers this hoping it would help them unpack their narratives.

Distress can originate from diverse sources: peer pressures, matrimonial setbacks, adolescence and advent of sexual changes, entering into a new institution – school or college, academic stress or defending a doctoral proposal, and/or death of a relative are sources visible in this book. It is response to distress which makes all the difference.

> *I was around 17 ... in second year college. You know it was the time when all the sexual developments are ... sexual orientation is changing. I came across a book by a Swami on brahmacharya (celibacy) ... There was a lot of confusion in me, and it produced conflict – made me violent. I could not study, I had to "drop" the first year of college.*
>
> – Jitendra, 60

Jitendra reminisces that lacking communication on the issue the sole option he had at the time was to read a specific book. The endeavour confused him further and developed in him an aversion for sex and sexuality. This was contradictory to his body changes and maturation. Consider the solid taboos associated with sex in the verbal switch he makes: *"You know it was the time when all the sexual developments are ... sexual orientation is changing"*. He switches his language from *"sexual developments"* to *"sexual orientation"* – a safer, socially more acceptable solution.

It appears he was experiencing a pull in opposing directions. One was his own body's signals, the opposite being a celibate monk propounding ascetic life, exhorting to ignore the body. Ordinarily young people discuss such issues among themselves, but there are some who may be socially withdrawn or too shy to discuss sexuality, especially if society considers it a taboo. It also appears that either Jitendra had no close friends or he chose to not speak with them. At a time when a young person needs to develop an understanding of their body, sexuality and the opposite sex, it appears as though (some) people work in an opposite manner – to instil in others a rejection, aversion and loathing for their body and its natural biology. A lack of communication made him feel as though his needs were arbitrary, socially unacceptable and possibly unnatural. By silencing the adolescent about something small yet bothersome, a whole apparatus works by suppressing the natural development of a youth. When sexual issues are not duly resolved do people become sexually troubled, or do they spontaneously resolve these issues? Perhaps this area needs future intervention among the youth.

Distress in academic milieus is testified by many narratives, each confirming how the experience of going through academic life itself can be stressful. The combined result of such stresses and individual subjectivity make people vulnerable. Parker et al. (in Barrable et al., 2018) note that students have a host of changes to manage, including making new relationships, living apart from friends and family, acquiring new study skills and learning to function as independent adults.

> *I had these symptoms for a long time. I mean, almost from the end of the third year of college. First of all, I could not study. While studying I would get so worked up that I would remain tense the entire duration of my exams. The way other people learn and memorize things in an hour, I would take forever ... With great difficulty I managed to complete my degree.*
>
> – Hetal, 24

In relating her distress, Hetal indicates that studying was burdensome and stressful to such extent it kept her agitated for prolonged periods. In addition, comparison with her classmates made matters worse for her self-esteem for she found herself lagging at something others did seemingly effortlessly.

> *I was 15 years old when I was given a diagnosis. When I was in standard IX I did not have sleep and I was continuously talking in the school, and failed in all subjects. My mathematics teacher wrote a letter to my mother asking her to take me to a psychiatrist.*
>
> – Vindhya, 44

Vindhya showed an earlier onset of deep anxiety, while still at school. Her agitation made her lose her sleep, which had consequences on her school performance. A teacher intervened and directed her and her mother to a psychiatrist.

> *My uncle just had a ... some breathing problem and ... that evening ... he expired, he just, he had a heart attack and he expired ... Yeah, it was a very sensitive thing that I went through. Then after that I had my class term exams and I couldn't ... my neck was also stiff so I had to relate my ... this .... my.... this paper to someone else and she wrote it down.*
>
> – Smita, 45

Smita suffered an emotional setback due to the sudden demise of a relative, which unsettled her considerably. Many a time, she mentioned the phrase "a very sensitive thing" to me in our discussion. She insisted it was something of great significance to her when it happened, for it impacted her school performance. In school exams in India, students who are considered "dis-abled" due to some reason are supported by volunteer "writers" who help them take their exam. The examinee usually dictates to them their responses to questions in the exam, and do not write themselves. If Smita felt so disabled by the death of a relative it goes to show it was not an ordinary experience for her: it had serious repercussions. To make matters worse she *had to* take the exams and was not allowed a postponement or exemption of the same.[8]

With Akshay, it was a combination of living with a partner amidst daily conflicts, malnutrition, academic stress and marijuana. When anyone is pulled in conflicting situations on multiple fronts, it naturally diminishes their ability to deal with any of them effectively.

---

8 This is a legal dimension, wherein a reasonable accommodation could have been made.

There were many factors ... one was a relationship. I met her in my first semester and we started living together. In my third semester we used to have a lot of fights, which began to drive me nuts. I was suffocating and would blame myself ... In my fourth semester I was introduced to psychoanalysis and I started seeing everything through that lens. So much so that I thought I was getting some deep revelations, which were not available to everyone. I was also smoking weed from the street, and there was a total lack of nutrition.

– Akshay, 30

The stressors mentioned here appear in many narratives with minor variations. School or college education repeatedly appears as a source of stress. At a time when a person is experiencing turmoil due to multiple reasons, there is also a lack of avenues for communication on the subject. Since young people need to talk it out to understand many situations, many aggravations can be diffused without going through any process of reification. Yet having no outlet they mostly end up talking among friends and peers. In every case, it is a cumulative effect of several underlying factors, never one reason alone which causes a "breakdown" or a rupture in the process of making sense of the world around.

It was one week before proposal defense, in front of the doctoral committee. High stress situation, as faculty were known to attack every potential candidate, and everyone wanted to be well prepared for that ... further funding to continue education in US was contingent upon that ... I reached my sibling's house at 2:30 am driving through the night (500 miles) with a friend, from Southern California, talking a lot, as though I had found some breakthrough theory to explain everything.

–Rupali

In Rupali's language, the metaphor of war is so evident that it immediately draws attention to the sense of imperilment she would have faced. A foreign location, potentially (or imagined) adversarial doctoral committee, impending loss of scholarship which she was dependent on, and the risk she took to drive down through the dark night. It appears as though all the pressures gradually coalesced into a "breakthrough" moment the rupture happened!

From a linguistic perspective, her language is replete with symbols which evoke a sense of insecurity, conflict at several levels, fear of self-preservation and sudden ability to take risks, as though there is a spiralling loss of coherence, pushing her to act and save herself. Seen in this perspective, Rupali found herself in a situation where her multiple freedoms

86

were compromised, her status marginalized being a foreigner, financially dependent and facing possibility of failure at the hands of the thesis committee, or possibly other issues. The issue of setting is crucial: *in front of the doctoral committee. High stress situation, as faculty were known to attack every potential candidate, and everyone wanted to be well prepared for that ... further funding to continue education in US was contingent upon that.*

Why should "doctoral committees" be so constituted that they invariably become stressors? Why ought senior scholars be seen as "attacking" rather than helping the doctoral students making their presentations? Why should a student's entire academic career, in terms of "funding", degree and possible jobs depend on a single presentation? This is a frightening scenario. The issue here is not that some suffer so acutely as to feel "helpless/ broken/ depressed" but how do other manage not to? Or do they hide it at one point to explode at another in future?

Ingleby (1980:60) points out that since by no means all who are placed in the situations we have described above become "mentally ill"; rather than leave the residue to be explained by vague and immutable "constitutional factors", it would be preferable to see whether the concept of interpretation itself could be modified to give it greater explanatory power. The central aspect of the interpretation I offer comes from the idea of social power, derived from epistemic privilege (see Chapter 2). In each of these cases, there is a deeply entrenched, relatively non-negotiable power imbalance, making each person a recipient of a system: a relatively inflexible structure which works mostly in a unidirectional manner, from the top downward. It does not have the pliability to respond to people's subjectivities, only a predefined framework all must fit into. The system expects conformity because non-conforming actors will only disrupt the equilibrium of a socially established system – school, university or work place. It is possible those who conform will move ahead, and minuscule others will fall by the wayside or get ejected out. Each person who experiences intense distress faces this prospect. To be inclusive society needs to create support for potentially vulnerable individuals.

But what is psychiatry's social power directed towards? What does psychiatry want to accomplish by the exercise of its socially mandated role? In response to this, as summation of the narratives above, the theme that emerges is "conformity". In each of these instances, whether Rupali, Akshay, Smita or others every individual is seen as doing something culturally "inappropriate". Therefore, they are referred to the clinic: to make "inappropriate" behaviours more "culturally suitable". In this context, Ingleby (1980:41) reflects that "[t]he social function of psychiatry can be summed up as the control of deviance; that is, the norms of mental 'health' and 'illness' are essentially matters of cultural judgment, although positivism misrepresents them as matters of empirical fact" (ibid:30).

But why seek psychiatric help in the first place and who is at the forefront of making this choice?

> *I was in America as a student at the time. The first dosage of medicine I got was in the US. But then we moved briefly to be in Delhi, because I was not well and during that time we met the doctor in India. Every psychiatrist was only reinforcing the other.*
>
> – Rupali

Cognizant of family history narrated by her sibling and later mother in India, both American and Indian psychiatrists were quick to implicate the "genetic factor" and attributed her sudden "symptoms" to a genetic predisposition. Both confirmed one another's "reading" of her situation, and the third sibling was a ready conduit to help confirm pathology. Centralizing a biomedical perspective, discounting her subjectivity, simply by looking at her behavior all actors first independently, then in a cumulative manner agreed that she was indeed "psychotic". Consider the pathos of "*Every psychiatrist was only reinforcing the other*". The adverb "only" is significant here; the expectation, a natural one, was that "the other" doctors would give different opinions and may suggest alternative routes for the person's predicament.

Jitendra had a relative who could guide his family towards seeking consultation.

> *My family members ... took me to a doctor. And somehow ... my ... one sister, cousin ... is a psychiatrist. So that may have helped my parents to know that this may be a psychiatric problem.*
>
> – Jitendra

A sibling or a cousin referred Rupali and Jitendra to a psychiatrist – both referrals made by people who were aware of the institution of psychiatry and symptoms of "psychosis" from prior exposure. Rupali's sibling knew due to their other sibling and Jitendra's cousin knew for she was a psychiatrist herself. It is clear that both sibling and cousin were not in doubt about their respective recommendations: there was certainty, a deliberation and comparison with existing evidence they were aware of. Both referrals and choices exhibit recognition of existing discourse and acceptance of need for biomedicine. Instead of any alternative, they straightaway took Rupali and Jitendra to psychiatric clinics. Neither felt a need to explore another path, look for a different explanation(s). A straightforward hypothesis was readily available and actions followed. Both Rupali and Jitendra exhibited submission and acceptance of this recommendation, doing as directed. Neither had an opportunity to discuss what was causing distress, yet both behaviours were *observed* by others, adjudged "abnormal" and the course of medication established. Notice that "patients" hardly go to the doctors on their own; they are usually *taken* there by others.

In a small way these outcomes respond to my earlier query as to why biomedicine becomes a natural choice, which happens in either of the following scenarios:

(a) Anyone having prior exposure to psy-knowledge: more likely to seek psychiatric explanation for people's distressed behavior, manifested as anger, violence, excessive talking or anything else;
(b) Having family history more likely to invite a psychiatric label, for psychiatrists are likely to attribute a genetic causality;
(c) Proximity to a psy-professional makes it more likely for someone's distress to be seen from an "illness" perspective, rather than offered a somatic or any other explanation.

The last is further confirmed by the experiences of Sona and Nithya both actively seeking psychiatric help for themselves. In contrast with Rupali, or Jitendra who were diagnosed by others, these young women did not wait for others to intervene. But they are also the *internet generation* looking for ways to deal with their problems online; in the process finding the discourse of psychiatry a befitting explanatory framework. Both had doctors in their immediate families, yet they were reluctant to pay heed to them or their recommendations, which may well be a sign of their independent decision-making capacity. They flagged their own distress as pathology, confirmed it by reading explanations on the internet and sought help directly. Self-diagnosing educated youth have a tendency for problem solving; they do not shy away from taking any path towards a solution. Scholar of rhetoric Fred Reynolds notes that in this age of self-care, websites like WebMD and commercial advertisements for depression drugs implore viewers to talk to their doctors about the specific symptoms, illnesses, treatments and adverse reactions detailed on the sites and in the ads (Reynolds, 2018:9).

> *All these years, I was without a diagnosis. In my first year of college I had too many thoughts in my brain, which were very bothersome. I told my father I needed to see a psychiatrist; there was one close to my house. When we went to meet her, she took a long time, almost six months, to decide whether I needed medication. Finally, between the psychiatrist and psychologist they decided. After thinking for many months, they put me on many drugs. My father and sibling (both doctors) were not keen to start with medication.*
> — Sona

> *Those days my father developed a drinking problem, due to pressures of a home loan. It became somewhat serious. In the middle*

*of the year I came home and the house was under renovation; I
felt terrible. I had come back from a hostile environment at college
and was looking forward to some rest; instead I was faced with
the mess around. Then my father decided to accompany me on the
way back, and in the night he drank on the train. I got very upset.
Once I reached my hostel, I kept getting into fights and brawls
with everyone. I told my parents I wanted to see a psychiatrist, but
they said no. My uncle who is a doctor said, "if you are not crazy,
they will ensure you become crazy by medicating you"!*

– Nithya

What is clear is neither had access to any helping professional at college, or
perhaps some distressing situations could have been mitigated. Both decided
independently to meet a psychiatrist, even while others discouraged them, and
in both their lives many others were involved in the decision-making process.
Conflict over whether to seek diagnosis or not came out from their narratives.
Their families were reluctant to consider the psychiatric route, they themselves appeared more driven in seeking it. Their attunement to the existing
social discourse, and education enabled them to read and understand from
the internet, helping them choose in favour of psychiatry.

In a third kind of situation, Hetal lived with her distress for years, and
managed to complete her college degree. Her father looked for help, both
for her and her mother. He did not refer to a psychiatric clinic as first option, though in time he did. When Hetal met the psychiatrist the conversation started with talking about her fears,

*He asked me, "[d]o you feel afraid", and I said yes, I do. I feel
afraid in my sleep, feel afraid at night. So he asked "do you generally feel afraid". I said yes, I generally feel afraid.*

– Hetal

Her father shared his own struggles having two people in his family to be
responsible for.

*Whatever we heard of, we went looking for it in every possible
way. We went to Balaji in Mehendipur, and many other places.
Almost for two three years we looked for all options. Then finally
someone among the Brahmakumaris⁹ told us to meet a particular
psychiatrist and that is when we took that route.*

– Mr. Mehta

9 Brahmakumaris are a religious sect of celibate Hindu monks and nuns, who also admit
families among their lay followers.

According to the biomedical perspective,

> [s]tigma related to mental disorders, lack of awareness in common people, delayed treatment seeking behavior, lack of low cost diagnostic test and lack of easily available treatment are the main hurdles in combating the problem of mental health in India. In addition factors pertaining to traditional medicine and beliefs in supernatural powers in community delays diagnosis and treatment.
>
> (Reddy et al., 2013:2)

Yet from the perspective of families, it may be remembered the medical perspective is usually not taken without circumspection or there is some resistance towards the doctor's verdict since

> [b]oth patients and doctors are operating within a pluralistic medical culture ... Consulting *tantriks* and religious priests and visiting healing temples emerges as a "natural" course in the family's help-seeking behavior. Furthermore, a patient can simultaneously be receiving treatment from a psychiatrist and a local priest or *tantric* without any apparent objection from either "expert" or any cognitive dissonance for either the patient or the family.
>
> (Addlakha, 2008:165)

Nunley (1998:319) was surprised to find that in northern India, families of patients are present and active throughout the psychiatric process. At every stage of the psychiatric process, families are instrumental in the decisions taken, whether in favour or against psychiatric medication, or what other alternative/s to explore. So it is entirely the family's decision, and there is an invisible power struggle, in which the family is frequently proactive in the interest of their loved ones. He further notes that, it should not be assumed that the psychiatrists ... in India are themselves entirely comfortable with the necessity of sharing so much power with families (Nunley, 1998:320). This also creates scope for having families where there is little or no insistence on psychiatric medication.

It is largely a parental response to their child's distress that makes them look for solutions, and reach the doorstep of psychiatry – directly or through a convoluted pathway. It becomes fitting to hear parental voices relating to the time of distress.

Parental response to children's distress

At first we were unable to understand how to handle it. Later we understood that parents will have to take a major responsibility. We were both concerned and thoughtful how to deal with it.

I focused on reading about pranayama and meditation, while my husband and son supported with understanding the medical part of it. Regardless of what other doctors had to say, we always had more faith in the words of my husband and son. All decisions were taken within the family.

– Sona's mother

Even though there were doctors in Sona's family, they were reluctant to refer her to a psychiatrist, while she herself appeared keen. Due to her insistence, the family consulted the psychiatrist. In an average family this is usually not the case, and the opposite scenario is more likely to occur. It is mostly another upon observing an "irregularity" of behaviour/s do members of a family seek help from trusted people. Such people can be different for every individual: some may approach a friend for counsel, school counsellor, psychologist, psychiatrist or anyone they think can help. Bindhulakshmi (2006:76) notes that family is the one important site where "mental illness" is first identified. Like every other health condition, "mental illness" also puts a strain on the entire family ecosystem and therefore it is pertinent to inquire, how do family members cope with it. Do all the members in the family get involved or bear with the tension of negotiating with the "mentally ill" loved one identically? Or how else do family dynamics play out?

Not only do families at times, in small or big ways, precipitate an onset of "psychosis" they often remain at the forefront of everything that follows. This is not to suggest that families are the prime causal agents of "psychotic" breakdowns. This is to imply that family scenarios are often replete with instances that can cause deep traumas, leading to unresolved problems which in time may become bigger and more complex. Even though Sona's mother and the rest of their family had one view of the matter, Sona felt differently about it.

After class 12th I was quite depressed and my mother would shout at me every day. I could not handle it. As it is, I am quite critical of myself but I could have done with a little acceptance.

– Sona

In the Indian setting, family remains the main source of social and financial support and also bears the caregiving burden of the patients (Sarin and Jain, 2017, Dalal, 2019). There is little doubt Sona's parents and siblings would have been extremely concerned for her. But her distress also invites another reading of the picture: the person experiencing distress is also powerless in the family due to her inability to play the role (medical student in this case) expected of them. This inability is compounded by the manner her parents handle her distress, for they are not privy to what the source of their daughter's suffering is. Neither the daughter feels safe or comfortable to share it. Yet in their own way, how they conceptualize it, they are doing all that is possible within their means to deal with the situation.

> *She felt some tension even while doing a master's degree in India, for there was an overall difficulty in the family due to our other child being so unwell. Rupali felt as though there was a problem in the legs ... she could not focus on her academics. We never explored the option of a psychologist then, so when she felt a need, she also chose to talk to the psychiatrist who the other child was consulting with. He never prescribed any medication, though she went and met him a couple of times.*
>
> – Rupali's mother

Rupali had a sibling being treated for a "mental illness" already. Therefore access to psychiatry was neither difficult, nor taboo. When she faced a problem she herself sought an intervention, even though it was not something to be worried about, nor did the psychiatrist prescribe any medication. Yet the proximity of a psychiatric "patient" in the family, especially sibling predisposes people to think of their own vulnerability in similar terms. From their study Greenberg et al (1997:235) also find that younger siblings taking care of an older one experienced significantly higher levels of subjective burden and stigma than did those taking care of a younger ill sibling. In families with pre-existing psychiatric histories the choice to seek psychiatric treatment seems obvious; not needing reconsideration. The consensus around the belief of "mental illness" is clear, seeking psychiatric consultation is routinized. In such a milieu, the discourse of psychiatry is well accepted and treatment options readily accessible.

In a different set of scenarios, where a familiarity with the medical discourse is not present caregivers indicate their struggles with access to psychiatric views in the first place or seeking intervention thereafter.

> *Over the years I have spoken to many caregivers and the one thing we all have in common in the beginning is the time we take to establish what is going wrong with the child who is struggling. Everyone takes a long route to understand that this is an illness, and now even when a caregiver is talking to me, I know what they would be saying next ... the pattern is so frequent that it is predictable.*
>
> – Smita's father

> *Her behaviour was odd and it went beyond ... my management, I couldn't handle her. Also, she considered me as her rival at that point ... and then she had all those behaviours, beating me up like anything and talking some nonsense words, not obeying and many*

more things so the symptoms were very bad. I didn't know what it
is. I could understand that something is very wrong with her and
she needs help, that's all we knew. Actually we didn't straighta-
way ... refer to a psychiatrist ... but a psychologist known to us,
a friend I had. After one or two meetings that person referred us
to a psychiatrist.

– Bharati's mother

When the caregivers classify suffering (seen as odd behaviours) as "illness"
they also appear relieved. It seems to exonerate their own culpability if any
could have been established. Not all caregivers are interested in meeting
other caregivers, but Smita's father is one of those who are. His dialogue
reveals the connections he has forged with other caregivers over the long
time (over three decades) he has been Smita's caregiver. Possibly his need
to connect with others is an attempt at making sense of his own struggles,
and supporting another wherever such help could be extended. I discern a
measure of confidence when he says how repetitive all stories told by other
caregivers appear to him; everyone's struggle has an identical pattern to
establish "illness".

But most parents are interested in looking for an explanatory framework
which can explain the distressed behaviour, not curious for the reasons or
uncertain to look for a way out. Even if it seems implausible their loved one
could become "mentally ill", the social presence of psychiatry itself legitimizes its claim and explanatory dominance. Using the cover of scientific
medicine, psychiatry has managed to become the leading legally chartered
profession for the management of misery and misbehaviour reframed as an
illness (Kirk et al., 2013:2).

When parents see an "oddity" in their children's behavior/s they are not
able to link it to their own parenting styles in any way. A child's developing autonomy is perceived as a "threat" by the parent who in a reversal of
roles projects it on the child: Bharati's mother says her daughter was "not
obeying" and her behavior was "beyond my management". Quite simply
the adolescent is expected to remain obedient, her life "managed" by her
mother. And though she said that her daughter was "beating her up" there
is little explanation why she did. I did not question the daughter about this,
because I was interested in her independent testimony, not comparing their
narratives with each other's, regardless of her mother's version.

One way or another, by consent or by consensus, an individual is referred
to the "system". It is notable that "the inevitability of social relationships
is in tension with the modern idea of autonomy and independence of the
subject from power relations" (Rebughini, 2015:1). On the one hand young
people strive to be independent, but when it comes to a behaviour which
stands out and threatens power balances within the home they quickly lose
their autonomy. Others step-in to guide matters as they deem appropriate.

This is the point where the aspiration of the young person unsettles the social consensus of power relations. Bharati's mother appears threatened by her daughter's behaviour, and desire to have her way (about watching a TV show). The parent-child relationship rests on an in-built dominance, and rather than encouraging the daughter to develop independently, her mother is actively engaged in "managing" every aspect of her life; making Bharati extremely lonely, something she mentioned many times in our conversations.

A parental response to children's distress when based on the medical model reveals three pathways. The first is a straight path to biomedicine due to prior familiarity with the discourse. The second a search for explanation from resources available around, which may include non-psychiatric options like faith healing, homeopathy and ayurveda. On the third road psychiatric diagnosis is received via first consultation or recommendation of peers/colleagues or some authority figures. Each of these paths lead to the same outcome: a psychiatric diagnosis. In each case, psychiatrists also create a verbal understanding both with the "patients" and caregivers. This happens in all other fields of medicine too but in "mental health" this one-on-one relationship with caregivers serves an additional purpose: surveillance. Yet, this list of outcomes does not exhaust all patterns which appeared from the narrative data. One response exhibited a marked departure from the above possibilities.

> *When we tried taking him to a psychiatrist, he made it extremely difficult for us to. My daughter, my wife, me and him were going towards the railway station to go see a psychiatrist. He just got off the rickshaw, went and approached a policeman telling him that these people are forcibly taking me to a doctor. It became a spectacle there and the policeman also told us that it is better to take him home, because he doesn't want to go. We brought him home, for it was clear he was adamant. After a few days we figured he was better and perhaps he could go back alone (to his university). All this happened in a span of ten days and after that he just went back.*
> — Akshay's father

The response of Akshay's father was no less unusual: he quietly observed his son's behaviour and let him have his way! And though the family did not push him towards psychiatric medication against his wishes, he himself chose it for a short time subsequently. There are a few noteworthy things in this scenario: first and rather unusually Akshay himself was aware of the counter-psychiatric discourse. Being at university far from home he was fairly independent and headstrong. But, the more important issue is that his family, no matter what their personal attitude towards psychiatric treatment, accepted his position and supported him in whatever other way they could. The attribute of *agency* is evident in a powerful depiction. The moot question becomes: when the individual wishes to exercise their choices, will the milieu, in particular the family, support it or obstruct its expression? Whether this creates a scope for recovery or further patient-hood seems a fairly straightforward outcome from here.

In the beginning of this chapter I proposed a three stage schema to explain the relationship with psychiatry. The segments covered until here are symbolic of the first stage of this schema: entering the relationship with psychiatry from different directions. Once the first stage is arrived at, the individual has entered the domain of psychiatric medication, the second stage sets in. This stage is marked by stabilizing the relation-ship with psychiatry, searching for alternatives, trying to find a balance in day-to-day life and restoring whatever can be while attempting to rehabilitate.

At this stage many enabling and disabling possibilities exist for every-one. Of these I principally investigate the domain of medication, family and marriage, education and work, social connections outside of family and the effects of stigma. This stage does not occur quickly, for those who accept the diagnosis take between a few months to years to find an optimal dosage. Along this span the family's continued role and the individual's personal agency matters significantly.

Stabilizing with the medical regimen

One of the key yardsticks of achieving stability after the initial diagnosis is to have a drug regimen that a person feels settled with, which facili-tates functionality in other domains of life. At this juncture some people by complying pliantly submit to the medical regimen, while doubtful others search for alternatives or a way out of the medical model. The willingness to stay within biomedicine may be seen as "the subjectivizing dimensions of the practice of adherence" notes D'Arcy (2019:95). Com-pliance with appropriate, recommended and prescribed mental health treatments simply means that a person is following a doctor's orders. Most patients are partially compliant (Bener et al., 2013:273). The rea-son for non-compliance may include "discomfort resulting from treat-ment (example medication side effect), expense of treatment, decision based on personal value, judgment or religious or cultural beliefs about the advantages and disadvantages of the proposed treatment, maladap-tive personality, traits or coping style (example, denial of illness)" note Roy et al. (2005:24).

Whereas from the point of view of psychiatrists all "patients" ought to continue treatments until told otherwise reality is doctors (mostly) *never recommend* otherwise. Going off psychiatric medication or even reducing dosage is often a complicated issue in a society like India, where psychiatrists believe that patients have to continue treatment until end of life.

> *The psychiatrist told me that without medication, if you play around, between taking medicine, not taking medicine for some time, you will never get better. To build up to the requisite dosage it will take three months because what you require as per body weight, cannot be given immediately as it will be toxic. It was weighing on my mind that this will all be expensive, and there was talk of increasing dosage. As it is, medicines made me feel sick, imparted a feeling of heaviness.*
>
> – Rupali

Here the psychiatrist appears to threaten Rupali she would "never get better", for she is seen taking her chances with medication. The former may possibly be threatened about his professional expertise for here is a "patient" not following recommended "treatments" with expected docility. By making the prognosis he not only establishes his epistemic dominance – knowing what the "patient" does not, but also warns of consequences for not following, namely *continued suffering*. Regardless of the "patient's" subjective truth: the sickness she feels or rising costs of treatment, which the psychiatrist neither asks, nor shows interest to know, he is forceful enough to convey his "truth". The patient takes it without further challenge to his authority.

When "patients" express their experiences of ongoing "treatments", psychiatrists often brush aside their testimonies as "subjectivity" and "non-scientific", even if they report feeling "sick". Subjects stigmatized by negative identity prejudices, says Medina (2011:16), may not be regarded as normal epistemic subjects, as reliable conveyers of information, and therefore they will not receive proper recognition in testimonial exchanges and will be unfairly treated.

It does not appear from the above dialogue what the "patient" reports is consequential to the psychiatrist; following the drug protocol seems his singular concern. Epistemic injustice in the case of illness can have devastating effects and can range from the subtle and hard to detect bias to brutal rejection of clear evidence of suffering (Carel and Kidd, 2014). The patient or her testimony seems incidental whilst "fixing" her symptoms paramount. Rupali is unable to express her side of the picture; whether expense, or the side effects. The doctor in his confidence and certainty does not seem to care enough to know that the patient has something more to report. Focusing on the epistemic dimensions of these situations Carel and Kidd (2014) aver that "patients" testimonies are often dismissed as irrelevant, confused, too emotional, unhelpful or time-consuming.

So while Rupali as "patient" is silenced by an epistemically outsized view, Sona's response to the same dominance is a stark opposite, as noted earlier. She herself sought psychiatric intervention due to the propaganda that *this* was the proper way to deal with her "problems".

> *I myself didn't quite fully believe in letting go of medicines but somewhere I always believed they will go. Even my mother used to always say that it will go but I never believed her, being so medicine oriented. Nobody ever knew how psychiatry worked. The only idea I had in my head was that I do not know how to handle this situation (that I could not study). I felt a need to go and look for a way out, to meet somebody who would be able to help me deal with my situation.*
>
> – Sona

Even though she was uncertain about the manner in which psychiatric medication works, but a discourse so embedded in society as solution becomes an obvious choice, in spite of her family's opposition.

Similarly Nithya initially showed a willingness to comply with her recommended medication. Yet she wanted to know the length of time it was required for. It would appear to be a logical query for if there is an "illness" there ought to be a "cure". But asking a psychiatrist does not evoke a straightforward response for most "patients". In a doctor-patient dyad it is usually the "patient" who is at the receiving end, for unlikely a doctor would agree with what a "patient" has to say, more so a woman. The omnipresent psychiatric discourse is reinforced by the peer group she is part of, whose goal is ensuring compliance and continuation.

> *If I ask him whether I'll be cured in five years of medication, he says, possibility of an episode recurring is reduced but cure is not guaranteed. My issue throughout has been medicine. Even in the peer group I went to, this was precisely what I said, while everyone else argued for compliance.*
>
> – Nithya

Rupali, Sona, Nithya are all educated women living in families who look at psychiatry with an independent view, often marked by ambivalence. Their doubts remain unarticulated due to the powerful and hegemonic discourse of psychiatry which silences every doubtful voice, shoring up volumes of evidence, while a majority of people do not have the ability to understand the nature of such evidence. Whatever misgivings they exhibit are nipped in the bud, and remain unchallenged due to what I refer to as *epistemic marginality* of "patients". Yet these women are not the average "submissive" psychiatric patient when it comes to questioning a doctor.

Now the following narratives represent those individuals who unquestioningly become subjects of psychiatry, conceding to its diagnostic control. Every other reality for them is secondary insofar as their "mental health" is taken care of by a doctor.

> *Oh yes, but he said that right now it will take you a couple of years. You stay on this course he says. So I think that once the doctor is managing the medicine I don't bother about it. It is okay, I am on medication ... Once I joined work this routine (of waking up, eating fruits, going to temple e.t.c) was disturbed and I started feeling the symptoms more because my office environment was stressful. Due to my fear the symptoms got aggravated and I had to refer to a doctor.*
>
> – Hetal

Hetal is better-off following her own routine, but work environment is stressful, pushing her into psychiatric refuge. From these testimonies it appears as though people are seeking psychiatric support to deal with their day-to-day issues – to study (Sona), to work in a stressful environment (Hetal) and to deal with tension (Vindhya).

> *I never tried to stop the medicine. When I am tensed or restless, my doctor will increase the dosage, when my tension suppresses he will reduce the dosage, or change the medicine. When the dosage is reduced I feel disturbed for about 10 days and after that I go with the reduced medicine.*
>
> – Vindhya

"Patient" voices are dwarfed upon their encounters with psychiatry's unified thunder. The institution of psychiatry maintains its dominance over everyone, though there are largely women in this study. Other social actors are engaged by psychiatry to ensure compliance to medication, though in this segment it may not be evident. In other locations the same women have reported this.

While people seek psychiatric help as a first line of action, whether they remain with psychiatry or look for other ways too marks the next stage of the process. The medical regimen may be dominant, but in a milieu where people also tend to be sceptical or open to plurality of views, they often do not entirely submit to the medical claim of pathology.

Searching for treatment alternatives

Usually when "patients", or caregivers question psychiatrists about duration of "treatment" the latter either respond by saying it would take a few years or openly declare it may last a lifetime. I call this a *stable* or *plateau* phase. At this juncture some "patients" themselves, or another in their family, may start looking for alternatives; even as a majority of others continue taking prescription medicine without questioning their efficacy, prognosis, long-term effects or duration. Those who do not agree with this line of approach start searching an early exit, as a few in this study also did.

> *I had left medication for several years – It was not as if anybody had told me to. It was a decision taken mostly on the advice of my husband, who said this is not required. But then depression symptoms aggravated, my moods were.... I mean there was irritability and all those things. At the time I was living in Calcutta, and I consulted another person.*
>
> – Rupali

People take chances with psychiatric drug withdrawal, especially if they do not feel relieved of their "symptoms" or if they do not believe in the conceptual framework of psychiatry. It may be recalled that Rupali took a Ph.D. degree while still on medication. She had a curiosity to look for other alternatives for her distress. Most publicly visible pathways lead to psychiatry, or *nowhere*. She chose the no drug option, which did not help at that time. One way or another she just braced herself and dealt with her suffering, searching between psychiatrists. Research evidence indicates that patients are increasingly looking for alternatives, especially in complementary and alternative medicines (CAM). There is global evidence about increase in CAM usage among patients of diverse sorts, including those with mental health issues (e.g., see Frass et al., 2012, Sharma et al., 2016, Thirthalli et al., 2016). Rupali knew about alternatives and tried a way out in whatever option appeared for the moment.

Sona had earlier said that her psychiatrist was reluctant to prescribe medication, so she continued to suffer in a different manner, due to her unaddressed suffering. Yet in response to her father's illness, she did not seem to exhibit what would be seen as an "appropriate" response by her own measure

> *During that phase my father passed away; I didn't cry. Instead I remained happy. I remember being in hospital looking after him, after his kidney transplant. I could not register simple things ... that my father was so serious and in hospital – he was hypoglycemic. My father died ... I told my mother that I need to get married. Then I thought this is strange and I went back to see my psychiatrist – she put me on anti-psychotics.*
>
> – Sona

This dialogue reveals the tremendous conflict Sona was facing: on the one hand an inability to register her father's illness, his subsequent death or an "unfortunately timed" urge to get married soon after his demise. She adjudged her behavior as "strange". Lacking what seems as though an "appropriate social behavior" and not following the "socially mandated" tropes of daughterly responses, she doubted her sanity. In judging them by a fixed yardstick of un/expected responses is a person not setting herself up for the social *ideal*, instead of following their own momentary truth, however absurd? Seeing herself not "responding" in a manner she was *expected to*, she castigated herself and self-selected "corrective action" via psychiatric intervention.

There are two contrasting behaviours to be considered here: one, an acceptance of diagnosis and taking on the "patient's" role and its polar opposite – ambivalence or rejection of the psychiatric verdict. In the latter case for lack of visible alternatives people continue psychiatric "treatments" yet do not stop searching for alternatives. In a third situation, on an opposite end of the spectrum, someone may be completely opposed to medication.

> *In my family there is a tradition of doing yoga and other disciplines. So they did not attempt to "cure" me immediately. One major decision was not to force psychiatric medication on me. They did not give in to social or psychiatrist's pressures.*
>
> – Akshay

To not cave in to social or familial pressure takes considerable agency. In Akshay's narrative his determination to resist medication is visible from the start itself. Yet without family support this may not have succeeded. Not only does family support his decision, they also shield him from rest of society disallowing anyone to meddle in his affairs. His father's testimony earlier also confirms this.

These cases exhibit people's search for CAM alternatives, while taking short-term recourse to psychiatric medication. But there are multiple factors which deter someone, for not only is there a looming psychiatric discourse there is also the question of social approval (for other alternatives, which are routinely demonized) missing in the overall environment. As a consequence, people are largely left to take their own decisions or "risks", if they dare – a bravado few hazard as "patients" or caregivers.

Relational aspects of recovery

Several kinds of relationships appeared in the narratives among members of the natal and marital families. There are relationships with psychiatrists, the wider world outside the home and friends or peers. For people living with families, the role of family in handling mental distress remains central. Pompili et al. (2014:2) believe it would be of great importance since the support given by relatives is an essential contributor to the well-being of the person/patient and a positive prognostic factor. Pathare et al. (2018:4) note,

> [e]xtended families in India play an important role in providing practical, material and emotional support to their family members with mental illness ... This reduces the perceived need by individuals for support from peers and simultaneously a discouragement by families to seek support from outside the family.

In numerous cases families tend to keep loved ones within domestic confines, holding stories of distress at close quarters. This attitude has different implications in different cases, with many variations which can be teased out for better understanding. Yet at the intersection of stigma and identity prejudice, this "closely guarding" attitude appears to have certain temporal advantages, which disappear in the long run. I will refer to this in the segment on stigma a little further.

Anthropologists Gammeltoft and Oosterhoff (2018:533) argue that mental health conditions are embedded in domestic worlds. The ways in which ill persons and their families imagine the future give character to their strivings and ambitions, shaping the choices they make and how they navigate the domain of everyday life (Sousa, 2016:47). These choices occur in every domain from treatment compliance to medical regimen, choice of career, marriage and other significant decisions. Mental "illness" diagnosis of one person has consequences for everyone, putting a strain on them, which "produces tensions within families" (Bradley and Ecks, 2018:1). Yet the same also carries a potential to exhibit "how kinship ties can take sufferers closer to acceptance and recovery" (ibid.). It must be recognized that family is not a homogeneous institution. Families can be vastly different in terms of their size, the relationships between members, intergenerational complexities and other attributes. There is also a marked difference between natal and marital families' responses. We may at best treat them as two kinds of families in which roles, expectations, pressures and challenges faced by the same person can be enormously different.

To examine the nature and outcomes of family support I asked my contributors two interlinked questions: what was their first encounter with psychiatry like and how did members of their families react to their seemingly "abnormal" behavior/s and its diagnosis? I distinguish here that this question further evoked two kinds of responses; parental versus siblings' responses among those who have siblings. Therefore, there is another subsection to document the nature of siblings' support. First, it is the reaction of parents.

Parental response

Parents do not always have answers to what afflicts their children. Yet their support or its lack makes tremendous difference. Citing the case of a woman from Brazil, Gammeltoft and Oosterhoff (2018:533) note that domestic conditions played a particularly important role in mediating how larger structural forces affected her mind and body, granting her certain life chances while denying others. This may be a universal reality. Domestic conditions make a difference for everyone, and changing domestic dynamics can enhance or worsen the prospects for recovery.

> *Initially the family had no other recourse but to follow the same trajectory they followed for my sibling – psychiatric medication. My mother came and supported me when I was in the US for my Ph.D. She took leave from work, and stayed with me … when I had to go over my thesis defense.*
>
> – Rupali

Consider the fact that Rupali had another sibling diagnosed "bipolar". When she showed similar symptoms in all likelihood it set the alarm bells ringing in the whole family, both in India and the US. At the time Rupali and another sibling lived in the US, albeit in two locations. It was this other sibling who conferred with their parents and took her to a psychiatrist, even brought her back to India soon after. The resignation of the family to accept Rupali's diagnosis seemed evident also in my dialogue with her mother. Yet, no matter what their initial response they did not hold her back from continuing her doctoral research. After a month of being in India when she was stable enough to resume research, her mother accompanied her, to help her transition from the setback into the flow of academic routine.

Jitendra also had a supportive experience; everyone in his family remained kind. Both his siblings being older remained cooperative to the best they understood.

> *I think it was quite good … means they treated me very nicely. Not only parents but … also sibling and sister … I think that was one of the important … point in my recovery. I mean nobody treated me in a bad way so there was no overall damage … I think they were basically cordial, cooperative.*
>
> – Jitendra

I noted earlier, Sona was herself keen to be diagnosed and medicated, even though her family discouraged her. Usually they let her decide for herself – whether she wanted a diagnosis, take medicine or try other options. Even talking to her mother evoked a similar response; nobody interfered with her decisions and she had full freedom to decide her course of action, on all issues. Possibly due to lack of communication on issues that troubled her she had no recourse but psychiatry's.

> *My father and sibling were not keen to start with medication. My father always listened to me, even when I would yell at my mom.*
>
> – Sona

Whatever the power of psychiatry in Sona's narrative its control over the family appears to be lesser than on the "patient" herself. In fact, her family encouraged her to look at other options or focus on her on-going medical degree. An opposing scenario played in Vindhya's life, both she and her mother believed the diagnosis and she meticulously followed medical advice. At the time we spoke Vindhya lived alone; her mother and sibling had passed away.

> *My mother supported me till she was alive. But today I have no one to take care (of me), in my family.*
>
> – Vindhya

In many families a medical prescription is taken as an edict. When psychiatrists enjoy such a powerful position nobody dares question them. What "patient" who stands in a queue to meet a doctor would dare ask them anything about their life or long-term prospects? Even caregivers are mostly fearful to ask anything, for everyone believes that the doctor "knows best" and working in their "best interest". Vindhya never questioned her psychiatrist and being a compliant, dutiful "patient" always reported her symptoms when asked, took another prescription and returned home. This had continued for nearly three decades when we met. By and large when "patients" and families seek psychiatric support they remain compliant automatically. Women remain more so and it is a lesser struggle to make them adhere to a prescription as compared to men and boys.

But Akshay's narrative had another unusual element: his parents letting him have his way from the start. After his father brought him home from the university where he lived at the time of his "meltdown", his whole family gathered around. His parents wanted to take him to a psychiatrist, but he resisted. He stayed home for two days, and then told them he would like to go back to university. They did not object to it. This brings a question of *agency* and the role individual agency plays in determining the life-course of someone's "mental illness". I will deliberate upon this ahead.

In many dialogues the ubiquitous dominance of psychiatric discourse stands clear, which both "patients" and caregivers submit to. Whatever conflicts or struggles within families, they do not seem to lie in the context of adherence to psychiatric drugs. The absolute social power of psychiatry, its "expertise" kept guarded within its linguistic boundaries, does not communicate with afflicted parties as relational equals – not even when "patient" families are doctors themselves. But this is only one of the trajectories.

The second trajectory appears with Akshay, whose agency is respected by his family, primarily his father. Not only is the young man opposed to psychiatric drugs once his family gets involved his father stands by him, letting him decide his way, does not insist upon medication, nor let anyone interfere.

> *I am alive today because of my family. When I told my mother that I was not in a "balanced" state of mind and I cannot handle things, she came with me for a full term to the university. She would not complain even though she went through a big ordeal, and my father gave her strict instructions not to have any arguments. Once she found "ganja"[10] in my pocket and forbade me from smoking. I would still hide and smoke.*
>
> – Akshay

In his case the dual power of a father's dominance and the unyielding temperament Akshay exhibited helped him, the rest stood by stoically.

> *My father was the decision maker. He went against social pressures.*
>
> Akshay

Ordinarily psychiatry is seen as an enabler of patriarchy, for it keeps the power of social institutions, particularly family, intact and in the hands of men. But when a man in his dominant position in the family, opposes the social force of a dominant worldview based on his own convictions he is able to oppose even a socially prevalent discourse. I am tempted to think if Akshay had been a woman would this have worked ? Would her father or family permitted her to reject the psychiatric option? If it had not been Akshay but any of his sisters would this have worked equally well? I have no answers to this, but at least a new possibility emerges: the traditional power of patriarchy played an opposite role. This maybe a benign or benevolent face of patriarchy if one could describe it so.

Participation of siblings[11]

While all peers do not have siblings, there also appears to be a difference in the manner siblings respond. Some siblings are actively involved, while

---

10 Marijuana.

11 Everyone shared about their siblings;whether boys or girls, wo/men. I am withholding gender information to ensure an additional degree of anonymity or traceability of peers in this book from family descriptions.

others remain indifferent and/or removed from the lives of their distressed brother or sister. Consequently there are differences in outcomes to mental distress among those with siblings and those who don't. Rupali, Jitendra, Sona and Vindhya have two siblings each, Bhavna has three, Nithya and Hetal have one each, whereas Smita and Bharati are single children. Their differences are as follows:

> *Nobody ever treated me as such (a sick person). I only checked myself (in terms of diagnosis) from the start of medication. My siblings believe that I can still recover.*
>
> – Sona

Parents appear to respond to their children's distress differently if they have one child, or more. Among the peers in this book a majority have siblings. Rupali's, Jitendra's, Akshay's, Sona's and Bhavna's siblings actively contributed to their lives. As Nithya's sibling is younger they neither appeared to play a role, nor appeared anywhere in her narrative and Hetal also has a sibling staying overseas,

> *My sibling does not live with us, they moved to the UK many years ago. No they are not part of our lives in any significant manner.*
>
> – Hetal

In some instances families appear close knit: even distantly located siblings are emotionally involved in each other's lives. Due to such affinity parents also seem less burdened, not solely responsible for all decisions regarding their distressed child. Recall that Rupali had another sibling with a similar diagnosis, also under treatment. When she got a diagnosis, in the US, the family did not react to another child getting the same diagnosis as calamitous. The third sibling also insisted later that their mother came to the US and stay with Rupali for a few months. Even though the family took recourse to psychiatric medication, they supported her tremendously when she needed to go over a critical phase of academic research.

> *They (referring to sibling in US) spoke to the (Ph.D.) supervisor who was quite supportive ... and took a decision to bring me back to India. Later they insisted to my mother that she accompany me when I return to the US, at least for a few months. My (under treatment) sibling ... would explain things in a different way and it was not medical, pathological views... could give alternative interpretations, saying that this is one interesting way of looking at it ... so that would help. [We had] lots of conversations around that. That was very helpful ... I knew there was an in-between path somewhere.*
>
> – Rupali

In every narrative the presence of other children made a difference to the confidence of the parents and the manner in which they approached and dealt with a diagnosis. Perhaps it also helped when parents hesitated other siblings would speak for their diagnosed brother or sister.

> *One of my siblings and the older (of the other gender sibling) were initially more supportive, while mother was not. She worried why all this is happening. The younger of my siblings and their family live in the same house with me and our mother. Initially their spouse ... I guess ... was scared for their children because I used to get angry, it all happened because of the medication. But now there is no such issue, we all still live within the same house, even eat together every day, though we live on different floors of the house.*
>
> – Bhavna

Her mother, who was initially uncertain how to respond to the "schizophrenia" diagnosis, got encouraged seeing her other children support Bhavna. Possibly it helped her change her perspective about the situation, which Bhavna also confirms

> *later she also joined in and sort of became my oldest buddy ... openly supportive.*

It appears that larger families exhibit greater resilience and interpersonal support to all members than smaller families battling distress. Not only do siblings support their distressed sibling differently they also appear to exhibit greater patience, understanding and desire to accommodate them than what parents can manage alone. Possibly it also gives courage to parents who are then not so traumatized by the "illness" of one of their children.

It may be noted that all these responses are coming from the natal family. Interestingly these findings appear somewhat contrary to contemporary psychological theory and psychiatric practice, which see a correlation between negative childhood experiences and "mental illness" as almost axiomatic (Addlakha, 2008:200). In these narratives negative childhood experiences do not make an appearance at least to the extent traditional theories postulate. I wonder if this is a sign of forgetfulness by those who shared their stories, or is it a lack on my part that I focused on the "illness" experiences in particular and not the entire life story of a person. Or did I not have the tools to map it adequately? Or is it that people did not see a continuation of their negative childhood experiences lead to a "psychosis" eventually? At least one thing becomes clear: notwithstanding professional constructions of people's "pathology" when people themselves narrate their lives they are more accurately able to identify scenarios of extreme duress.

107

And, they inadvertently have, vastly different constructions from the so-cially dominant "expert" views about them.

Marital families

Marriage plays out differently for men and women with a "psychosis" diagnosis. For women the adverse impact appears greater. Possibly it is because women's suffering arises not only from biological and psychological dysfunction but from deeply conflictive gendered engagements with their life worlds (Sood, 2015:168). Whether or not this statement means "biological" in terms of "biochemical" the way psychiatry constructs it, the female endocrine system has a completely different effect on women's mental health, especially the role played by the thyroid gland (e.g., see Kamble et al., 2013, Bathla et al., 2016, Rakhshan et al., 2017).

Barrett (2000:460) suggests marital history influences mental health. How natal families deal with it is different from what unfolds in marital families. In the latter the emotional support a "patient" may get is not to the tune they are offered in natal families. While natal families often share responsibility of caregiving, in marital homes not only is this safety net suddenly gone, a woman is also expected to fulfil all expectations of conjugality and femininity. Epidemiological literature does not testify to the benign effects of marriage on women's well-being (Addlakha, 2008:201–202). My findings confirm the setback; in two forms. Rupali had shared her diagnosis with her partner-to-be,

RUPALI: *"I did not realize that marriage itself can bring on a crisis".*
ME : *"Then marriage is not a solution?"*
RUPALI: *"No, it's not a cure, because I also felt that maybe this loneliness whatever I am feeling – this depression that I am feeling, maybe it's a lack of companionship I am feeling ... it's not so easy. Marriage is a whole institution by itself. It's got its own life, momentum and families enter ... (it) gets very complex, because people have expectations. Even the initial highs of wearing those new dresses ... it all dies down after a while and you reach a point where you realize that if you don't feel good inside, then the demands of all this ... are just not making any sense".*
ME: *"Do you think marriage worsened things for you?"*
RUPALI: *"Well, I mean ... obviously pressures of marriage are there ... I think by and large you can say it worsened the situation because if you don't get to find a way out and you are looking for a cure, but you end up getting married then it's a very problematic thing."*

Initially her husband was supportive and discouraged use of medicines saying, *"these issues can be overcome with family support"*. But after their marriage, when it came to disclosing the same to her in-laws, he did not support her by explaining the situation to his parents. Neither did they openly discuss with her what the issue was.

> *In-laws knew about depression, but they never expressed anything openly or whether it was a problem for them. I could not even tell them that I already had an abortion and two miscarriages while in the US. Husband was not interested in having family but things changed after return to India, as pressure for maternity surfaced unexpectedly. Village women started insisting you must have a kid. (There was) sudden pressure from villagers and in-laws ... and I could not explain my husband was not interested! I wanted to move around and befriend people in the village, but the social position of the family was dominant and accordingly the perception. So I realized that I was just being watched. Soon being in the village was no longer a comfort.*
>
> – Rupali

She refers to the gaze of society or family over a person, in her case an outcome of a difference of social class. Being an urban woman she married a young man whose family lived in a village, while they were both in the US. Her words imply a woman is expected to perform class and gender-appropriate behaviours, which she experienced in her husband's village. Notwithstanding the confidence her husband expressed while alone with her, when it finally came to dealing with parental expectations he simply backed off, which became a source of tremendous stress for her.

Vindhya got married through the matrimonial sections of a newspaper. She was working, earning, felt confident about herself or her prospects ahead. Upon a little encouragement from her psychiatrist she took a decision to get married. Due to her new found self-confidence she did not share with her prospective husband anything about her diagnosis. When he found out later he could not take it in a stride.

> *Marriage was a total failure for me. Once my husband figured out that I took tablets he started harassing me ... he didn't beat me or anything, but he spoke very harsh words. He said that I had fooled him and questioned me "why did you fool me only, why me" ... made me very depressed. I even took him to my doctor later, and the doctor said you should try for a child.*
>
> – Vindhya

Citing M.J. Fields' research done in the 1930s, Ghana, Luhrmann (2016:8) notes, "that the stress of marriage could precipitate the illness". In both these women's lives matrimony brought back "symptoms" they had successfully dealt with, for it brought into their reality the in-built expectation of conjugality and progeny. If someone is on psychiatric medication, they are ordinarily recommended to go off medication for the duration of their pregnancy. Rupali had already discontinued her mood medication earlier, so

> *I felt I had a need to tell her (the gynecologist) I was bipolar. When she heard it she said, 'Oh ... you have to get it treated. **It cannot go on like this. I will stabilize you on the gynecological medicine but you have to take the ... mind medicine. It has absolutely no connection and with the pregnancy ... it is absolutely essential in order to get pregnant.***
>
> *So I went to a psychiatrist and he was very particular that I should take the medication. He kept telling me that you could cope with a certain amount of depression, **and now, until you come to your dosage, which is adjusted to your body weight, your symptoms will not improve in a marked way.** So I followed a path of increasing the dosage of drug for about four months. There weren't any major improvements except my appetite had suddenly shot up and I rapidly gained a lot of weight.*
>
> – Rupali

As Rupali had acted from her discretion without consulting an "expert" she was referred back to one by the gynecologist, whereas Vindhya was told to reduce or eliminate her medication to ensure a "normal" child.

> *When I went to the gynecologist she scared me that **if you are taking psychiatric medicine the child will be born mentally challenged.** On her own she reduced my medicine by half. I did not talk to my psychiatrist about it then. Once I reduced medicines which had helped me remain calm and carry on my job, I could not continue working. I had to leave my job.*
>
> – Vindhya

The fact that marriage and family are necessary stressors in the lives of Indian women has been noted by psychiatrists (Addlakha, 2008:245). The highest rates of distress are observed in the reproductive years, a period in the life cycle that coincides with marriage and child rearing. Marrow and Luhrmann (2016:199) cite Nancy Scheper-Hughes from her 1979 book wherein she "saw ... a social world in which people were consistently made to feel small and ineffective by others – parents, siblings, leaders, popular opinions, doctors ... (those) belittled and socially insecure were more likely to develop schizophrenia". From the two narratives it appears their symptoms were clearly exacerbated by psychosocial factors (Sousa, 2016:49).

Identical to the narratives Sousa studied, the narratives of Rupali and Vindhya also leave one to wonder if they would even have become sick at all if
after being married each had a more understanding husband ... and an elder
sister who didn't become terrifyingly ill (Rupali had a similar sibling) (ibid.).

In marriage a woman with a "mental illness" is likely to become more
vulnerable in a patriarchal society. In India social power is ordinarily tilted
away from women, in matters of disabling conditions it only veers more so.
Bordo (in Ghosh, 2018:102) confirms patriarchal power and the gaze construct the female body within different sociocultural contexts and power/
knowledge discourses by representing female embodiment as inferior to
male embodiment. As a consequence of systemic practices borne by such
belief, "[i]t is known that legal cognizance of mental illness can nullify con-
tracts, marriages, capacity to hold and manage property, custody of children etc" (Dhanda in Nagaraj, 2015:51). The W.H.O. (2000) takes note that
women's health is tightly linked to their status in society, broadly improving
with greater gender equality and exacerbated by discrimination. Mathias
et al. (2018:2) cite several studies suggesting gender inequality is a key determinant of the differences in mental health between men and women.
Where marriage does not create a symbiotic balance between spouses there
is greater likelihood of adverse effects on the mental health of women.

The need to connect with others is a basic human need, and marriage
is only one way for it. People need social connectivity for myriad reasons,
many of which foster their well-being and health. So what happens to those
who are unable to create such links and become isolated? In what manner
can their isolation further complicate their lives as psychiatric subjects? The
writing that follows looks into this.

Far from others as "bounded beings"

In an astute description of the fundamental estrangement that can be someone's lot, Gergen (2011:7) introduces the idea of "bounded beings" as a way
of being which keeps people apart from one another, except in a self-serving
manner. Underscoring the need for relationship as the hub of human life,
action, social being, ideas and further, Gergen questions

> [w]hat if we could understand all that we call thought, fantasy, or
> desire as originating in relationships? In the idea of the "bounded
> being" he centralizes the notion of human estrangement and how
> people "celebrate autonomy", the "self-made man," the individual
> who resists social convention and marches to his own drummer.
>
> (ibid.)

By this depiction he highlights that because people remain so self-conscious
and self-serving they remain fundamentally alienated from one another. As

111

an outcome of this attitude they remain bounded within their mental and emotional walls as though to protect themselves from one another, circumscribed within boundaries. Thus they become isolated and progressively lonely for the separation, suspicion these walls build create deep fissures of mistrust which are difficult to bridge.

I extend the idea of the "bounded being" to contexts of "mental illness". In particular it brings to mind those who live fairly circumscribed lives. Instead of a life in the midst of relationships which can provide scope for social integration they face a state of fundamental estrangement from the world around. In such a situation the individual has a limited number of people to fall back on and connect with. Such connections then usually remain confined to parents, who also happen to be caregivers. Eventually the whole family becomes burdened and careworn with the exercise of looking after the "ill" person. This cyclical and mutually reinforcing scenario creates great eddies of suffering. Both "patients" and caregivers are tied to each other in a grip which they cannot loosen; it seems to choke them all.

ME: *"How far is the editor you report to?"*
HETAL: *"The editor is in Bangalore, we talk on the phone when there is a need for it."*
ME: *"Okay, you do not go out to meet anyone?"*
HETAL: *"No I go, I told you ... weekly".*
ME: *"Once a week you leave your home, that's all?"*
HETAL: (laughs) *"Once a week yeah".*

As a young person given a "schizophrenia" diagnosis Hetal lives with her parents. She appeared fearful and socially isolated. The limited semblance of social networks she has created lie in a spiritual practice she volunteers for. Yet she tries and goes out independently.

> *So what I do for that is that I organize courses (for the spiritual practice) ... That way I get to meet other volunteers on a weekly basis.*
>
> – Hetal

People look for meaning and social connections in many ways, even by organizing groups of diverse sorts. Whether it helps them socially integrate is a different issue, at least it does not leave them socially marooned. Becoming socially isolated is often *not* a personal decision or choice. It may reflect others' behaviours or response towards them, which "patients" do not know how to deal with. In Bharati's narrative a case of fundamental isolation appears more starkly.

I am very lonely till today from the time I was 15 and ... when I went to my 11th standard it was a great shock that no – none of my classmates they talked to me.

At the time of my conversation Bharati was 22 years. Her situation had not changed much. We spoke several times and she mentioned about her lone-liness on every occasion. Her social ostracism continues for no reason she could identify. She feels people either find her behaviour odd or deliberately avoid her, even if she tries to befriend or invite them over. Her mother's version of the story made the picture come together in a different light.

We lived in a joint family. His parents were with us and also my sister-in-law's two children ... brought up in our family. I used to nicely manage everything and never sent her for tuitions anywhere because I – I am good at mathematics, (I am a) science teacher and ... language and all. I don't require any help from ... others for her education. I ... myself am an educationist. So I have spe-cial methods of teaching science and all these things ... I used to spare time for everything because my timings were well planned from 4:30 in the morning to look after my work, domestic work. Our's is a very orthodox family so ... for many years we didn't hire a domestic maid to help ... as long as I was healthy. Only when my mother-in-law fell sick and I developed a cardiac problem we could hire a domestic help.

– Bharati's mother

This is the context which she raised her only child in. Living in an ortho-dox joint family puts tremendous pressure on working women. She tried to balance many sides of her domestic and professional life. Yet there was a cyclical pattern of control visible here: the joint family controlled the moth-er's freedom, disallowing her from employing a domestic help, whilst she herself had the means to pay for it. She, in turn, controls the freedom of her child in another way – by keeping her close to herself in all academic mat-ters and setting her goals. It has another impact – circumscribing Bharati's social relations or possibly most matters in her life. If a person creates im-aginary or actual boundaries around themselves do they not progressively become isolated?

Friends means not very close ones, and one girl was friendly with me and she used to ... as I didn't do well ... used to make fun of me, for everything .... I guess ma'am it is an important reason why they (all) avoided me. She used to come home and I think ... possibly she told other students something – something was wrong with me, and they didn't talk with me either. Actually she used to

come to our house and her parents used to observe us (as family)
a lot while they were nearby. I think she told others maybe she is
not alright ... "loose" (in) her head – that is "mental" like that she
would have told like that and till today they have avoided me.

– Bharati

There are several dynamics visible in this family scenario oppressing each person differently. There need not be any control when it comes to a child's academic outcomes, for control can be stifling. But here everyone seems to judge others by academic performance oriented yardsticks. Bharati's reflections on her classmates' views about her reflect the prejudice against someone unable to achieve acceptable standards of academic performance. Yet this is not all.

Considering her mother is an academic she has little trouble teaching the daughter most academic subjects Bharati needs help with. Seen from a parent's point of view there is no problem. But seeing from another perspective the mother ends up making herself the centre of Bharati's life: controlling most aspects of development of the daughter's selfhood. Ordinarily parents send their children to school and then expend further efforts in either teaching them or sending them for private tuition classes, to seek help for additional study. Not only did Bharati's mother rearrange her life to meet domestic responsibilities, but without realizing she ends up thwarting every opportunity Bharati may have to mingle with her peers. Progressively Bharati is left with no friends willing to engage her or visit them. The mother takes over further areas of her life, no doubt due to her intention of "helping". She therefore frowns when the daughter asserts herself to watch a TV program (noted elsewhere).

(Regardless her performance her mother told the teachers) *"Bharati*
must to go to the next class along with her friends. Any failure and
all ... will not help – me to recover her. So if you could do some-
thing more ... My request to her teachers proved successful as she
was doing okay in school. With just a minimum of E grade in all
subjects, she was promoted to 12th class. In 12th she showed very
good improvement. In fact, in accounts she stood second in the
class. So then at university stage we applied for Economics and
also philosophy ... in both she got admission it was purely on en-
trance basis ... we chose the one with no mathematics! I used to
support her morally. I also read up many philosophy subjects to
say so – because I have given her the confidence, which may also
be wrong to some extent ... now I realize ... if I go to my mother
and ask for any help ... she is there to help in anything ... So that
kind of confidence and relationship I have built with her".

– Bharati's mother

114

In her words there is triumph – over the circumstances of her daughter's life, an indomitable spirit to meet the goals and targets set for the young woman, pulling her along to accomplish them, regardless of the daughter's volition. The biggest challenge from the young woman's perspective is her abject loneliness; academic accomplishments mean but little.

> *Madam I have no friends to talk to. I am very lonely ... until to-day, there are no friends, and nobody talks to me.*

My heart breaks every time[12] I hear this. She follows her mother's recommendations dutifully, whether she tells her to study or do anything else, never asserting herself. Yet for the mother, she must be still "managed": engaged in one thing after another, not having the freedom to be by herself, travel, go anywhere alone, even take a local bus,

> *Perhaps you would understand ... she is a simple-hearted, inno-cent girl. If I let her travel by local bus some young boys can get after her and say irrelevant things to her or worse ... you know how the world is after all. Then we have all sorts of people around, we are ... high caste ... !!! I think you understand all that, no?*
>
> – Bharati's mother

In an interlocking pattern the young woman is disempowered by various social institutions, all acting simultaneously to completely enfeeble her. Her "high-caste" birth and university-going status are not enablers to rehabilitate. Instead they become sources of further oppression and ensure she remains *obedient and docile*. In no decision for herself she can exert freedom. All her goals and choices must be decided by her family, every movement monitored, watched and guided by in/visible controls, whether they come from biomedicine, parental guidance, the caste system or lurking rapists that she has to be saved from. After all, she is the "girl child" – always girl, always child! And why not, when the same apparatus which had to facilitate her movement from girlhood to womanhood is choking her every effort towards self-expression, why would she not remain a "child"? She remembers the fateful episodes of hitting her mother, and out of that shame concedes to taking medicine. What can she do but submit to external controls and continue feeling guilt for actions from long ago? Her mother continues giving her medication for *that reason alone*; nothing else she accomplished ever since counts! The circle perpetuates unperturbed.

---

12 As I said in Chapter 3 my connections with several peers continue for years and I remain connected to them via different channels, including Bharati who appears off and on.

I asked her many times how she felt, how her "symptoms" were. She is fine, and in the course of time that I interacted with her,[13] she moved from doing her first to a second master's degree! The fears of her mother to let her go out independently, rough it out like young people her age, look for a job and travel independently seems to be a key factor in her decision to take up another degree instead of a job, or anything outside the university's "safe" environment to which she can travel with her mother. Her experience seems to coincide with the anthropological evidence offered by MacGregor (2018:6) that people judged as mentally disturbed and considered vulnerable and dependent would have less control over their movement than other adults. Is she actually all that vulnerable, or is she believed, or even made, to be vulnerable? Is this belief of her vulnerability out of concern only, or reflects a (parental) temperament that basically cannot trust anyone? There is no way to tell. But it leads me to a related question – if a young woman is considered so vulnerable in what manner would she overcome her real or imagined vulnerability and lead an independent life, if not in her early twenties?

Bharati's world is tiny: bounded within frameworks established by her family. She does not question them, for who knows whether further questioning or rebellion invites censure or re-negotiating "dosage" with the psychiatrist. To make the young person conform to parental authority, ensure compliance and docility the whole apparatus operates as though through an invisible hand, which guides the process. In this manner she remains "safe", the colonizer lurks within.

I draw upon the conceptualization of *social capital* by Robert Putnam (in Morrow, 2001:38) as consisting of social and community networks; civic engagement or participation; community identity, involving people's "sense of belonging" to the community, and norms of co-operation, reciprocity and trust of others within the community. Bharati entirely lacks social capital and it brings deep sadness. As a young person cut off from everyone in the world her world is constituted only by her parents or ideas in books, and academic degrees. From her work in community mental health in Uttar Pradesh and Uttarakhand, Mathias (2016:xvi) confirms that people with mental illness also described experiences in their communities and families of discrimination and social exclusion. Most encounters with "mental illness" seemed to lead to impoverishment and reduced social capital.

> Theoretically, social capital in the context of health-related research attempts to link micro-social individual behavior and macro-social structural factors ... Health behaviours and practices may superficially appear to be a private matter for the individual,

---

13 A span of nearly four years.

but in reality health practices take place in a range of social are-
nas, which for children, are constrained by everyday contexts,
which will vary from school/institution, family, and peer group
and neighbourhood.

(ibid:39)

No matter what stage of adolescence or youth, this estrangement has been a
significant part of her experience – in school, at the university in a five year
degree and then another master's. Jarman (2001:4) notes that sociologists
frequently emphasize the ways in which social exclusion is better viewed as
a set of processes as opposed to a fixed state. Seen from a social exclusion
perspective, Bharati is socially excluded whether by choice or its lack. The
scenarios which create her exclusion do not change – they continue across
her life (as of now). Is there a way this estrangement could be bridged, and
who can support that? By all yardsticks she is an educated young woman,
yet without agency or willpower to question any dominance. This confined
living, with minimal interaction with the world is an internalized behavior.
How would she ever forge a relationship with any person her mother hopes
she would someday? What sort of a life can she expect to have as an adult?
The web of relationships that can enable and assist socialization can also
have an opposing outcome. This irony is evident in her situation.

Though families can support "patients" by becoming enablers towards
recovery, it cannot be overlooked that families can also be key sources of
distress. Many a time family scenarios can be oppressive and dominance-
oriented. They can suppress the emergence of autonomy and agency of the
individual. But there can be other ways too in which agency may be compromised, as another example illustrates in the next segment. Suffice to say
that education or academic degrees do not suffice to empower if someone's
family believes it to be the sole way to rehabilitate or recover. Until education creates social inclusion and facilitation for the individual it means but
little. Such one-sided education, wherein she can only take one degree after
another serves only an instrumental need: to garner more degrees. When
will Bharati mingle with the world, take up a job any degree has imparted
her skill for or meet others beyond the family's protective shield? Though
her educational enterprise leads her to more degrees she only grows unilaterally in the intellectual domain. Consequently she gets further isolated
from all opportunities to interact with others due to parental over-concern.

Rehabilitation and its outcomes

Recovery, defined broadly, is not only the remittance of symptoms, but also
the process by which people are able to lead productive lives that include
working, learning and participating in their communities (Sousa, 2016:49).
When people enter into a therapeutic relationship with psychiatry they do

not remain confined to their "patient's" role, though in exceptional cases that may happen. Mostly people try to reconfigure their life in ways that accommodate their newly discovered vulnerability to stresses and create a life by factoring them in. Yet, how best to encourage people in their recovery process remains a pressing social and clinical question (Myers, 2016:428).

The steps towards recovery begin with rehabilitation efforts, created in many stages, built on one another progressively. These stages work as building blocks helping someone climb to a certain level, enabling them to make a leap into a new, *healed* self – the recovered self. For Slade (2010:2) recovery is seen as a journey into life, not an outcome to be arrived at. Narratives of people who have recovered from serious "mental illness" emphasize the centrality of hope, identity, meaning and personal responsibility. No matter what stage, people muster the courage or enabled by others to meet with their goals and challenges, attempting rehabilitation to whatever extent feasible. In this process three options appear.

Getting up after the fall – continuity amidst transitions

Once the initial heat of the moment passes and a path discernible to contain "psychotic" *meltdowns*, often via psychiatric medication, it is time to restart life. This is the turning at which everyone behaves differently. Some give-up the stress producing situations entirely and chart a new course, some carry on with the old course to complete the incomplete, unfinished project/s and others completely abandon all effort and fully take on the "patient" role. This difference in responses produces three different outcomes, in time. A majority of the peers in this book continued whatever they were doing when derailed by their meltdowns.

> *Mine was a theoretical research and by the end of one year I was quite stable. I made weekly visits to a counselor, and monthly visits to psychiatrist. I managed the Ph.D. this way. After that I did a post-doc as my professor created the position, for eight months.*
> – Rupali

> *I started doing activities, started ... attending classes, college.*
> – Jitendra

> *My mother was there with me during this phase, when I returned back to the university, as I had told her I cannot deal with all this by myself. All those problems went away slowly. But I continued having anxiety, cyclical thoughts, trying to prove to my girlfriend that I was alright and I had done nothing wrong. This lasted for six months. Slowly I came around. After finishing my master's degree, I became okay and returned home.*
> – Akshay

118

In the year after my graduation from the medical degree I could not get any option to pursue a specialization, so I took up a job in a hospital in the skin department, which got over in August. I stayed home for another six months.

– Sona

I was given a (schizophrenia) diagnosis when I was 15 years. I completed a bachelor's degree in Electronics and Communication later and went on to take up a job. I even worked until I was 30. Then I got married and it produced different complications.

– Vindhya

I will soon be finishing my MA degree too and then I am thinking of either joining a diploma in French or may be a Ph.D. degree. I am not sure yet, still thinking what to do.

– Bharati

At the time Bharati told me about this ambivalence she had still to take a decision. But in the preceding segment I have already noted how in fact she chose to take up another master's degree. All these people returned back to complete their on-going degrees, seeking help from available resources among which the role of family is apparent.

Course-corrections

Nithya felt the stress of the on-going degree and scenarios unfolding around too much to deal with. She left the degree after her meltdown without completing the degree, towards a less threatening option.

I could not continue with my engineering after the first year, and left. Instead I entered a program in sociology. The doctor recommended continuing medicine till the end of graduation. My mother thinks I stopped taking medication before the end and therefore I had a second breakdown.

– Nithya

Hetal managed to complete her degree yet discontinued further pursuit in the technical field she had trained for and chose writing instead, which facilitated dealing with her distress differently.

I used to write on a blog I had created. I would translate spiritual texts like the Ashtavakra Gita, and listen to Guruji's commentary about the same. My mind would feel a lot calmer with that, I felt

119

markedly improved. Only after that I had taken up the job. But since the job ... my blog-writing was reduced, and later I could not write at all. In fact my psychiatrist ... he was surprised that I could take up a job. I mean ... he said, "oh, you do a job, very good. You are coping well".

– Hetal

Notwithstanding inability to deal with the pressures of their situations, it is noteworthy that neither women discontinued making feasible efforts. By duly recognizing their situational stressors they even switched pursuits. At the time we met (separately), both were taking some doses of psychiatric medication. They were ardently exploring other options as well, their respective parents also shared. In fact, both sets of parents spoke with me extensively in-person, as I met both in their homes.

From my perspective the comment of the psychiatrist to Hetal appears to be *patronizing*. It appears from his words that a "patient" would not be expected to take up a job, is seen incapable of doing anything and certainly not expected to be socially or financially independent.

Bhavna joined work in her sibling's construction company. She adds,

I was working with them but ... because of my ... skin allergies and infections I had to stop because the doctor told me not to go out too much in the sun, heat and dust. Then I started a small catering enterprise of my own, taking orders for meals and so forth.

It is evident these women corrected their course wherever required to. It shows a certain cognitive flexibility, and ability to think/ act rationally, identify stressors and take independent decisions which enable further growth. Neither of them required constant guidance or supervision from others.

We talk about schizophrenia as a single disease, but in fact, recent research suggests that the illness likely consists of a group of disorders with heterogeneous etiologies, rather than one circumscribed disease entity. That schizophrenia manifests differently and to different ends in different people.

(Sousa, 2016:48)

A search for the "best" treatment as fighters of "schizophrenia"

At times a person may become so troubled by their experiences they become less than functional in several domains. They try to adjust to their diagnosis and continuously search ways to deal with it. Smita also deals with her life thus, with active participation of her father, though her mother was also active in the past. Smita tried many rehabilitation options including computer courses, working with non-governmental organizations, etc. Her father became problem-focused as his daughter's schizophrenia label appears to have disturbed him deeply. He took her from one city to another in search of a "cure", and not finding it in one location, looking for the next possible destination which would get them closer to their goal. One can imagine how they stressed themselves in this process. It would have been a big hassle going from place to place, doctor to doctor, and starting all over again in different cities. Recounting about her experience at a prominent psychiatric rehab facility, where she spent the better part of a year, she says,

> *I had a bad time there. I had to put in lot of hard work. Like, you know I was into baking, grill, cakes. Yeah, it was very difficult for me because I was going through a very ... you know I was very down. Even moving on to that one baking job or candle making, soap making, pottery and stuff, it was ... it was really tough to learn. The fact that I had to walk so much to the ... to the activity centers that was just another torture for me. I couldn't, I had to just drag myself to the center where the baking was going on.*

Yet this effort at rehabilitation in an institution of *significance and repute* (her words) did not produce any meaningful consequences. For Smita over three decades of "treatments" has only meant a change of city, scenario or day-care routines different institutions put her through. Each helped organizing her time in one activity after another, while life has remained more or less static. There is no fundamental or transformational change. She meets with her psychiatrist regularly, meticulously follows the drug regimen, and reposes tremendous faith in psychiatry's methods, including the wisdom of her psychiatrist. Overall the stable narrative remains stability-focused.

Among all contributors to this study, Smita is the only one who goes into day-care for the past decade. She is one of six peers with a "schizophrenia" diagnosis in this book. Two others have a history as long as her but her life has turned out rather different from theirs.

> *Five days a week I take a bus ... and return home by 5 pm. The whole day is spent there, doing various things like computers, cookery, teaching, etc. I teach ... once a week, and on another day I manage some office work.*

When I ask her about her life, future and other prospects she rues,

"We are fighters of schizophrenia, not survivors."
ME: *"What does that mean?"*
SMITA: *"I think it means that there is no hope for them. I mean there are people who are survivors, may be you are among them too. There is hope for you, but there is no hope for the likes of us."*

Her words stun (and pain) me, for not only she is aware of the social category of "survivors"[14] she also believes that they (we) have better prospects than those struggling with their diagnosis not finding a way out. She is insightful enough to know,

"Survivors, you can say, they can have a future. But ... what I am trying to say is that I don't think anyone in this institute can proceed further".
ME: *"Oh, why do you say that?"*
SMITA: *"I think it's just activities (in this day-care) and such things are not enough, I think counseling could really help."*
ME: *"Is there no body coming for counseling?"*
SMITA: *"No, but they have their doctors."*

Many thoughts occurred as I pondered upon Smita's words over time. The issue of her agency resembles what was visible in Bharati's narrative. Ingleby (1980:41) calls this process self-reification, noting it as the "very essence of mental illness: the patient ceases to experience his life as meaningful and himself as an agent, and as long as the doctor remains in the positivist framework he can do nothing but encourage this self-invalidation". It is also clear that these women never get a chance to ask about or intervene in the decision-making process about their own medication (Bindhulakshmi, 2006:114). Smita knows whatever rehabilitation could have occurred within the scope of her day-care center has been accomplished. There is an awareness of possibilities outside the center but options to access them are limited. Her fate is decided between her psychiatrist and her father. No matter what a nod from the psychiatrist is always important for her. Without that approval she lacks the courage to strike out on her own and her father does not permit anything outside day-care.

My dad has to be convinced, he is just not ... you know he is not giving in and I am really getting desperate now.

At the time she shared this Smita was 44 having a three decade "treatment" history. That she is/was unable to convince her father is evident, and until

---

14 Which not many people in this study were aware of, until they met me, whereas I never personally use this word to represent myself. I was unaware of this social category the entire span I took medication.

he agrees she cannot do what she wants. But what makes her father so firm? Is it the belief in her schizophrenia, as though it sums up her entire life? No doubt "the tag profoundly colors others' perceptions of her (him) and her (his) behavior" (Rosenhan, 1973:181). The invisible hand of psychiatry determines future trajectories of her life just as it does Bharati's.

Earlier I had indicated about Bharati viz a viz. a fundamental estrangement from her milieu. She has many attributes in common with Smita. They were both given a schizophrenia diagnosis (at nearly 15 years each), the first social setback they had to deal with. Their narratives depict how "practices of informal social control prevailing in the domestic sphere" (Addlakha, 2008:117) render them without agency and absolutely powerless. This lack of agency does not manifest only with regard to their treatment regimens but pretty much all other life choices. The fourth issue is that they have no one to speak for them, as support from siblings is a foreclosed option; both being single children.

The fifth common factor is the response of their respective caregivers to their diagnosis and their relationships with psychiatry.

> Meanwhile I also started reading lot of literature about the nature of that (schizophrenia) because, I didn't have much knowledge ... research articles and all, those things. So I knew when we used to go to the psychiatrist what will be the course of action.
> – Bharati's mother

Living with a schizophrenia patient can put considerable burdens and restrictions on the rest of the family (Jungbauer, 2004:665), leading to increased stress and subjective burden for caregivers (Mathias et al., 2018:16). For the average educated person who is capable of reading any psychiatry-related literature, the likelihood of reading ideas of this nature is completely natural, for it is psychiatric knowledge or literature which dominates the milieu anywhere, more so in the internet age. Bharati's mother is a highly educated person and to find, read and believe psychiatric research is easier for her than to read the counter research questioning psychiatry. Her self-directed *continued education* about prognosis of the "disease" becomes an aid for psychiatry: it helps ensure compliance to medication.

Response to stigma

Crocker et al (in Link and Phelan, 2001:365) indicate that stigmatized individuals possess (or are believed to possess) some attribute, or characteristic, that conveys a social identity that is devalued in a particular social context. What is not so well understood is how stigma impacts the day-to-day functionality and reality of a person. How/does it damage their selfhood and imperil social integration in a society prone to prejudice, due to the stereotype associated with the stigma? More so, "[r]esearch examining the sources and pervasive, socially shaped exclusion from social and economic life are far less common" (ibid:366).

Three aspects of stigma surfaced in the course of this analysis: (a) how people look at others due to stigma (b) how the person themselves self-stigmatize or internalize the stigma of a stereotyped social category and (c) how in a self-reinforcing rigmarole they isolate themselves irrevocably, making recovery more complex? Livingston and Boyd (in Firmin et al., 2018:1) confirm that consequences of internalizing stigma can be severe, and report associations between internalized stigma and increased symptoms and decreased hope, self-esteem, self-efficacy, social functioning and treatment adherence for those with prolonged "psychosis".

Link and Phelan (2001:363) review the work done in understanding stigma, ever since Goffman's seminal essay (Goffman, 1963) and affirm the negative impact of stigma on the lives of the stigmatized.

> *I was withdrawn, and would not talk to anyone. People saw me as 'ajeeb' (strange), as I would sleep during the day ... so sleepy that I would sleep between lectures, on the sofa in the common room. And I did it multiple times.*
>
> – Sona

Whether or not someone said anything to her, Sona appears to have internalized the stigma and believed that people perceived her as "strange". In a school or college environment everyone wants inclusion in the peer group. Being apart from one's peer group can be humiliating and stressful. Stigma affects social interactions, social networks, employment opportunities, self-esteem, depression and quality of life in general (Link et al., 1997:177). A stigmatized individual becomes immediately vulnerable to pre-existing social schemas (Smith et al., 2011), silenced and their social exclusion due to the stigma becomes an additional source of distress, in addition to the label.

> *I used to feel sleepy in class ... everyone was asking what is the reason for sleeping in school. At times I would go to the back of the class and sleep ... I used to feel shameful when I woke up (giggles) and everyone would be looking at me. One girl asked me "why are you sleeping like this". A couple of them asked me more seriously and maybe to one or two I revealed something about memory tablets ... something like that. Then ... she told me not to take those medicines and said "that's why you are sleeping so much".*
>
> – Bharati

When classmates look at them questioningly it is often not possible for someone taking psychiatric medication to share the truth. But even without saying so their behavior is perceived "unusual". Ever since this phase of her life, Bharati got isolated from her peer group, as nobody could understand her suffering or sleepiness. For anyone dealing with side-effects of psychiatric drugs, social isolation and loss of social capital is a harsh reality. The inclusion and connectedness they need to rehabilitate and create a space for themselves as a social actor is denied by the milieu; few have patience for someone whose behavior follows misunderstood cues and markers. Thus, a self-reinforcing rigmarole continues making the psychiatric reality wellnigh an overarching truth, a self-fulfilling prophecy.

At times people may seek validation of their choices by looking at celebrities who are increasingly talking about their mental health conditions around the world, as exemplars of "illness" labels and advocates of medication. But Nithya dismisses that stigma is reduced because of celebrities.

*Celebrities can do anything and it can become acceptable. But stigma is still there among lay people. Having traits in common with celebrities makes people feel better about themselves.*she says astutely

Notwithstanding perceptions, in some families "mental illness" remains a well-guarded secret. It is never shared with those outside the "circle". When I went to meet Nithya's parents, they were so guarded at first that they worried our conversation may be overheard by their next door neighbours. Only upon assurance I could talk to them freely. Similarly, another family kept the diagnosis within close doors.

ME: *"Nobody got to know (about your diagnosis)?"*
BHAVNA: *"Nobody got to know".*

This practice is prevalent: nobody ever talks about anyone's "mental health" issues outside of domestic spaces, or beyond trusted people. It appears to be a useful strategy for keeping matters guarded so no stigma about a person's (vilified) identity gets perpetuated. Research on stigma documented discrimination against persons with mental illnesses in housing, jobs and social interactions (Mann and Himelein, 2004:185)

> The labeling and stigmatization of a woman as "crazy" begins within familial and social spaces and, over a period of time, leads to her removal from society into seclusion ... Stereotypes about "mentally ill" women (as incapable people who need to be forced into treatments) abound in many non-custodial institutions as well ... "Institution", then, is not just a physical structure but also an attitude or an approach towards people that can be found in all kinds of places.
>
> (Davar, 2015:3–4)

These narratives make it clear that every family shows a different response to stigma. While a majority of people choose to remain quiet to avoid further stigmatization, some do not see their children from the points of view of a devalued identity, whereas some totally believe in their labels and deal with them with a "custodial" attitude, even though their children are not in any visible custody. Among these narratives the caregivers of Smita and Bharati believe in this form of custodial care, entrenching further their daughters' status as *women with schizophrenia*.

I analysed peer and caregiver narratives to unpack psychiatric subjectivation using a critical discourse analytical framework; an effort to understand how distress morphs into a diagnostic category. My goal was to see how social power plays out during the subjectivation process. I have lain in front of the reader how a person in distress is referred to a psychiatrist and from where begins their "sick role".

5

FROM SUBJECT TO AGENT *OR* WHAT IT TAKES TO RECOVER

> People tell stories not just to work out their own changing identities, but also to guide others who will follow them. They seek not to provide a map that can guide others – each must create his own – but rather to witness the experience of reconstructing one's own map.
>
> (Frank, 2007:17)

In this chapter, the open ends left behind earlier come together. Unlike the quote above, while this writing is not a self-narrative yet in sharing with a peer and via me with a wider readership, these narratives are afforded a scope for re-telling, re-interpretation and a new synthesis, helping us all get closer to the goals of this book. In the previous chapter, I investigated sources of individual distress, the process of becoming a psychiatric subject and myriad catalysts that assist subjectivation. The numerous relationships one is embedded in contribute towards reifying subjecthood or depart from colonization. Not everyone becomes a subject for their remaining lives. Their circumstances, personal dispositions, co-morbid conditions, a critical mind or even the presence of a chance person who guides the process can lead to freedom from subjecthood.

Recovery in no part of the world is a straightforward process. In a country where a vast majority is unaware of such an option, the degrees of complexity are more tangled. When the milieu itself is information deficit, whatever enablement could have come from the macro-environment is not available to anyone. Therefore, anyone who recovers after a short or long stint with "psychosis" stumbles upon the process, not knowing whether the choices they make are leading them toward or away from recovery. Only at hindsight can we comprehend the outcome and its path. In the midst of it while facing various uncertainties nobody knows which path would lead where. Due to this uncertainty, there is an even greater need to bring these stories to light. They giveaway how seemingly random sequences across

DOI: 10.4324/9781003248804-7

narratives contain common patterns revealing unexplored avenues and possibilities. My attempt here is to map those patterns.

To or not to be, a subject

Perhaps nobody chooses to be the psychiatric subject they become. It occurs due to the presence of others whose chief role is insistence on psychiatric medication. In certain instances, subjecthood can be established more easily than others – visible in Rupali's and Jitendra's narratives; both having prior exposure to psychiatric discourse and professionals. Akshay on the other hand is an exception though also aware of prevalent psychiatric discourse. Uncharacteristically, he was also aware of the counter-psychiatric discourse. Such people are not present in large numbers anywhere, more so in India, where the discourse countering psychiatry is not easily audible, accessible or lies in the public domain for ready reckoning. Therefore, Akshay-like individuals may be the tiniest category. The other sort of individual is more easily found – aware of psychiatric discourse or believing it, not resistant to embracing psychiatry or its prescriptions. Such people become willing "patients", then subjects. In trying to find succour they are so keen to embrace a solution they easily believe the notion that being on psychiatric medication is in effect the path of being "in-recovery".

This belief also rests on the reality that clinicians propagate around the globe with a focus on clinical recovery. "Patients" overlook the fact what they require is not just clinical recovery but actual exit from drug dependence; prolonged psychiatric "treatment" itself is pathology. Although factors affecting prognosis with regard to clinical recovery are well known, the contextual factors facilitating this form of recovery are less explored (Bjornestad et al., 2018:2).This is yet another clinical view of recovery. In a dichotomous representation of the phenomenon of recovery, those who experience the subjective outcomes of medication want to be completely rid of them, for medicines bring tremendous side effects (e.g., see Healy, 2012, Breggin, 2013, Kirk et al., 2013, Gøtzsche, 2015, Whitaker, 2015). Accepting medication, in no matter how small a dose, serves as a constant reminder of one's "patienthood". Only once medication has been left behind, and the ability to deal with day-to-day minor or major crises developed do people really consider themselves recovered. The psychiatric version of being "in recovery" does not appear to resonate among those who contributed to this study.

Two distinct categories of people emerged from this study: those who are recovered and those recovering while continuing as "patients". By "patient", I do not necessarily mean incapacitated, but someone following a medical treatment regimen. In psychiatric parlance, we may call these two groups as people who "recovered from" psychosis, as opposed to people who are "in recovery" (see Chapter 2). Between recovery and "patienthood", a spectrum of possibilities exists for everyone, having several stages of rehabilitation, which build on earlier stages either progressively or simultaneously. Once several such stages are crossed and stabilized in a cumulative manner, one can make the crossover towards full recovery, by the manner of recovery identified in this study. It is notable, however, that these stages do not represent a fixed template that everyone has to or does follow; they are a broad schema, whose finer details vary in every case.

Recovery as goal: psychiatry-led or self-determined?

The recovery model, wherever it is propagated as part of current mental health policy or advocacy, is premised on the notion that recovery would primarily be a psychiatry-led outcome, patients would in all earnest follow the recommendations. This view gives the impression as though the option of people's recoveries due to their own abilities and capacity for problem solving is either foreclosed or does not exist at all. The following statement is a confirmation of this attitude:

> there is growing evidence that supports the contention that taking part in social, educational, training, volunteering and employment opportunities can support the process of individual recovery. People with severe mental illness need to be supported to create their own recovery plans.
>
> (Jacob, 2015:118)

By this measure, all options a person requires for recovery are already defined. So now the professional only has to assist the individual choose among them! The subtle message is that people, *obviously suffering a deficit of judgment*, need assistance in judging. They do not have their ability to make such strides on their own. Instead, they wait to be guided by their psychiatrists, not only in issues of mental health and its "treatment" but also in all aspects of life. These could be related to educational, vocational, financial, marital, child bearing or other social goals. The benign arm of psychiatry truly appears to take on a paternalistic role – not only can it "treat" a person's affliction but also "guide" them appropriately on how to live a "meaningful" life; an attitude widely prevalent in the Indian psychiatric community (e.g., Kulhara et al., 2009, Shields–Zeeman et al., 2017).

Such paternalism is not confined only to matters of guiding and supporting "patients" but also towards guiding public policy towards increasing psychiatric infrastructure. This is based on the view that more psychiatrists per capita be made available to the general population, which is said to remain underserved in matters of mental health.

129

It is often claimed, not just in India, that in order to promote mental health, the development of infrastructure, personnel and services should be given greater importance than the will and preference of the persons receiving the services; that questions of choice and preference can be addressed after a robust system of mental health care has been established.

(Dhanda, 2016)

Of late, the Global Mental Health Movement (GMHM) is another step in consolidating the treatment orientation in "mental illness" and attempting to change government policy and expenditures towards further increasing psychiatric infrastructure (Sharma, 2019:12). In other words, if there is a good enough mental health system in place, whose contours are decided and planned by the professional psychiatric community, there is nothing more to be done because people can then easily be taken care of by professionals. There is no question of whether society can work proactively to reduce psychiatric morbidity (see Chapter 7). We only ensure that people are taken care of *after* they are made dysfunctional or fallouts their incongruous personal contradictions produce! Clearly, by these criteria, mental health can only be addressed if there are enough psy-professionals around since there is no felt need to look at mental health early enough to prevent its deterioration. Consequently, there is only going to be a growing "treatment gap" (Kaur and Pathak, 2017), considering the size of India where we do not even have adequate healthcare. To have a further specialized mental health care will always fall short of its desired targets in such a big country, or anywhere. This is precisely the rhetoric of the GMHM while few question what outcomes "treatment" brings.

What are the mechanisms in public health science – in particular, epidemiology – that enables groups to sanction one account of disease causation over another, that is, to achieve monopolies on truth? How do such groups achieve the authoritative status to set public health agendas.

(Richardson, 2020:5)

From these views, it appears, given a multivariate requirement, diversity, complexity, compounded by inadequate infrastructure, especially trained psy-professionals recovery cannot occur. Such attitudes signal the colonial stance that until certain conditions exist the "poor barbarian" is not capable of problem solving, least of all related to knowledge. Not only does recovery have to be determined and regulated by psychiatrists, in most cases

well-meaning practitioners often agree in principle with this goal, but suggest that it is not yet the right time, or that we do not yet

have the requisite means, to achieve it. Their patients are too sick
or disabled to recover; there is not yet an adequate evidence base to
support recovery.

(Davidson et al., 2010:185)

Clearly, anywhere in the world, psychiatry takes it upon itself to lead the
process and point towards the direction of recovery.

By measures of this deficit orientation, people are *not* expected to exhibit any measure of agency,[1] curiosity and resilience of their own. In a
"patient's" dependent role and act of surrender, they ought to continue remaining so until their psychiatrist gives them a nod to think otherwise. No
doubt this attitude is conveyed to a majority of people who continue taking
medicines regardless of efficacy, hoping in the next pill laid the panacea.

The truth about recovery also reveals another picture. In the same manner
that the phenomenon of recovery appeared in its earliest evidence in the US
in the 1970s (see Chapter 2) with one person at a time recovering, such recoveries are now also beginning to appear in India. Knowledge about recovery is based primarily on the individual stories and resulting insights of those
with lived experience (Deegan, 1988).The complexity or randomness of the
phenomenon seems peculiar because there appears no pathway or certainty
which individual will or will not recover. So for now, these may be seen
among the early testimonies outside the psychiatric gaze. Such outcomes are
self-directed, happening due to people's search for solutions, their scepticism
of mainstream medicine and/or an ability to look for alternatives, a part of
the human temperament, especially in (medically) pluralistic locations.

> Recovery narratives are diverse and multidimensional. They may
> be non-linear and reject coherence. To a greater extent than illness
> narratives, they incorporate social, political and rights aspects.
> Approaches to supporting development of recovery narratives
> should expand rather than reduce available choices. Research into
> the narratives of more diverse populations is needed.
>
> Llewellyn-Beardsley et al. (2019:2/31)

In my sample of ten peers, there are three who met the "recovered" criteria
from the beginning: Rupali, Jitendra and Akshay. In each case, the role
played by psychiatry was different. Rupali switched out of psychiatric medication with the aid of a homeopath and other support, Jitendra was supported by a psychiatrist cousin and Akshay opposed the psychiatric option
from the beginning. He was supported by his family in dealing with the

---

1 Jones et al. (2016, p.1) define agency as the subjective sense of control or authorship over
  a given action or behaviour.

distress or pressures he experienced. The role of family, one's own agency, a continued search for alternatives, following a life course towards recovery and rehabilitation, and successfully dealing with stigma appear as significant parameters contributing to recovery in these narratives.

Beyond psychiatry's gaze – gaining autobiographical power

When a person's identity is transformed into a "patient's", there is a something akin to a loss of autobiographical power over one's self narratives (Myers and Ziv, 2016:397), which has an impact on mental health recovery. This loss of power, due to epistemic injustice (Fricker, 2007), is confirmed by Carel and Kidd (2014) as an outcome of identity power that psychiatry enjoys in comparison with "patients" it implicates as "mentally ill". Recovery, on the other hand, is a reversal of this loss. I propose this process as *gaining autobiographical power*: regaining the confidence, courage and ability to choose one's options without further guidance by a benevolent, paternalistic psy-professional and/or caregiver. It amounts to gaining the ability to deal with one's life challenges and no longer be a victim of *social defeat*. I draw on the ideas of autobiographical power and social defeat from Myers and Ziv (2016). These anthropologists describe autobiographical power, or power over the self-narrative, as key for mental health recovery.

Recovery stories, or first-person narratives of recovery, highlight the ways people return to a good life, sometimes even a better life note Myers and Ziv (2016:396). Whether or not people are able to return to a good or better life is a complicated question because it involves many degrees of assimilation and efforts at every level in society. Yet, this is the goal with which this chapter sets out towards further analysis of the three narratives where the narrators accomplished drug-free personal recovery and remain stable for years. I investigate key departures from psychiatry-led versions of recovery they made and how it impacted them in the short and then long term.

Before proceeding, I address the challenge to the idea of "Recovery Narrative" as a genre within mental health utilized in specific ways to promote the idea of recovery that Woods et al. (2019) draw attention towards. They analyse the form, function and effects of the "Recovery Narrative", calling it a highly circumscribed kind of storytelling.

> The lack of consensus over the definition of recovery, combined with an ongoing debate about whether it is or should be a "top-down" policy directive or "bottom-up" survivor-led programme of action, has focused considerable energy and research capacity on identifying and isolating its constituent components.

Since this study is by an ex-patient who has herself overcome psychiatric "patienthood", my goal via these narratives is also that in "telling an individual story ... (I) voice a wider political framing of mental health" (ibid). At this point it may be recalled that in countries like the US and UK, there is already beginning to appear a resistance to the manner in which recovery is implemented as mental health policy, whilst India is far from it. Therefore, the narratives I report do not serve the purpose of shoring up the agenda of psychiatry-led interventions at all. Uncharacteristically, I work with the idea of recovery using narratives as "a rhetorical device to unite interlocutors in their mission ... and (for) political persuasion" (Woods et al., 2019).

What does recovery feel like at a subjective level, and what are its attributes? Are people who identify as recovered the same as those who are "in recovery"? If not, what is the difference between them? I respond to these questions by analysing recovery as a day-to-day, strength by strength, incrementally achieved lived reality, not a theoretical, medical or anthropological concept. For this, I do not seek the opinions of "experts" about "patients", but relate directly with peers. Our recovery frameworks emerge from the experiences of our lives and narratives.

Recovery is not an idea or construction that everyone connects with in principle, as a goal or outcome. All three people who I classify recovered in this study do not find a personal resonance with the word at all! Yet they were accommodative enough to support my usage of it. They also accommodated my framing of their recoveries in the framework I proposed.

I try mapping this move from a psychiatric view of suffering to a non-pathological view of understanding the struggles of living. It encapsulates developing an ability to handle day-to-day life stresses, the chief reason why psychiatry takes control of people's lives. Those who move out of diagnostic self-constructions are better able to respond to daily stressors as they transition from "patienthood" to *selfhood*. For them whose "patienthood" is their first identity, most stressors overwhelm, producing anxiety. They tend to remain fearful and unable to either become or remain functional in most domains, whether professional goals, meaningful relationships, living independently, have social connections, marriage or family life. There are clear and sustained recoveries and *on-going* recoveries; the latter mostly drug dependent. Even those reconciled to "patienthood", a hope and dreams remain that things may change someday; though their own capacity to actualize it may be missing.

Discourse and recovery

The rest of this chapter is in two parts. I begin by looking at the impact of discourse's recovery. Thereafter I examine the meaning of recovery for the three peers I classify recovered, who have healed in a drug-free personal sense, not the psychiatric definition of clinical or personal recovery. This gives an opportunity to delve into factors that contribute to their recoveries. I also revisit the narratives of two caregivers of the three individuals, with intent to understand the manner they supported their loved ones towards recovery. Since the third person, Jitendra's caregivers (when he needed them in that role) are not alive at present I interviewed him without their inputs.

Looking beyond discourse

Given the complexity associated with the word recovery, asking someone whether they view themselves *recovered* appears brutish. Everyone has a different response, depending upon their age, belief in "mental illness" or recovery. At times when an experience is from years bygone, people may have an entirely different perception about it in the present than the manner they experienced it long ago. To suggest the word recovery makes little sense after years have passed unscathed. The actual experience of being labelled or psychiatric support is not part of their reality for years (even decades). The ideas around the theme recovery offered by all three recovered people do not resonate the word recovery (as though recovery from "mental illness") back to me! Their constructions sound different.

> *Yes I am out of all of that ... doctors, medications ... I have understood what it is. I have understood also my own behavioral triggers and things, so I know I have recovered from whatever it was, and I know how to deal with it. For me that is what the recovery is. Basically it is all about self-understanding ... Even if there is an imbalance, food imbalance or whatever. But I know when I am angry or something, I know there is a way for me to get back. I know it is temporary and I can get back.*
> — Rupali

> *I don't think that I am a recovered person. I don't connect with [it]. The past is over; it does not cling to me.*
> — Jitendra

> *The recovery part is that there are moments when I mentally really go down, and feel it is really quite terrible. But I come out of it also. And I know ... almost there is knowledge that this is not going to last – this state of down-ness of whatever, it's going to change. I have come out of it so many times now that I have started to feel the temporariness about it. Whereas, earlier it used to be that when the gloominess used to be there I had to make a herculean effort to come out of it and I would just go sliding back down into it. That's the difference now, it's just reversed.*
> — Rupali

Akshay does not relate with recovery word – "*recovery from ...?*" he shrugged.

His conversation is not diagnosis-oriented and there was no point discussing the issue further. His conviction disparaging psychiatry dismissing its labelling is not easily gained, for it does not rest on an ignorance of his distress. His evident self-confidence evinces agency based on knowledge he is convinced about, not whimsical youthful subversion.

In each of these expressions, whatever its form of enactment: rejection of psychiatry, distancing from its framework or outright dismissal, there is an effort to look beyond a psychiatric conception of life, suffering and meaning. "When our talk is psychiatry-resistant or even psychiatry-free, we do something very different, potentially even revolutionary. Simply by how we speak ... we are either tacitly upholding or undermining psychiatric rule" (Burstow, 2013:82). Neither of these peers is an anti-psychiatry activist, like activist-scholar Bonnie Burstow whose sentiments they seem to typify. Their spontaneously chosen self-representations are what she opens up a possibility for towards a radical change in self-conceptualization beyond psychiatric categories; an act of reclaiming oneself.

People inherently have a capacity to look beyond psychiatry if they are not wilfully made to follow its prescriptions. But how many really get those opportunities within their families and the social milieu? What could be the path that may lead to this change? Is it only about labels and nomenclature or is there more to looking beyond psychiatry? In the previous chapter, I narrated how most individuals continue taking steps for rehabilitation even after their diagnosis, yet not all recover fully. There is something extra which people do to recover, different from others, which marks their exit from psychiatric dependence.

Factors contributing to recovery

Recovery is a multi-dimensional, on-going outcome. Many contributions come from the external environment and several from self-directed action by someone herself. There is a multiplicity of directions one could look into to understand recovery from an individual's subjective perspective. Among the motifs in these narratives, the role of families seems salient in every case. The nature of family support makes all the difference between continued "patienthood" and recovery.

Another attribute of recovery seems to be age; most recovered did so well within their twenties and thirties. After crossing the age of 40 years, either recovery does not appear as an option most "patients" actively pursue or they have already given up. Every recovered person in this book belongs to this demographic. I do not believe recovery would not be possible above 40 years, yet this data indicates most do not actively pursue the goal.

Exiting psychiatric dependence

"Patienthood" starts with medication. Before medication, odd behaviours remain unnoticed or non-pathological until a psychiatrist steps in suggesting morbidity. So what role does medication play in the lives of those who recover? My question about continuing psychiatric medication has important other trajectories, linked to the search for alternatives. Though relatively little is known about how people subjectively experience antipsychotics, Larsen-Barr (2016:7) has investigated the attempts at drug discontinuation or the role psychosocial factors play in recovery outcomes.

> *You cannot interact with many (people) as things that had meaning earlier, no longer meant anything. Fortunately I had a counselor in the US who was very supportive, and who almost spoke nothing, but constantly listened. It was a great vent as there was nowhere else to talk. I couldn't talk so much even with my family, as they were in India.*
>
> – Rupali

The presence of counsellors and therapists usually helps someone express their distress if the therapist is not overly diagnosis-oriented. Larson-Barr (ibid: 35) confirms that some forms of therapy can serve as appropriate alternatives to continuing antipsychotic medication. Borg (2007:50) agrees that "[e]veryday life tasks need to be addressed as part of the practitioners' agenda, as well as if not more than such issues as psychic insight or medication compliance".

ME: *"So finally your cousin finally decided one day **that okay no more medicine for him, he is okay?**"*

JITENDRA: *"Yes, I mean for the last part of my treatment, the last two or three years I used to ... I understand that medication was started just to reduce the depression, and other things. So ... in last two-three years medication was started for that".*

These are two different kinds of responses, both mediated by professionals. A supportive counsellor and a psychiatrist in the family helped these individuals to view themselves in other dimensions than focusing on their "patient" status. If someone in distress gets to speak at that moment, it can be an effective venting mechanism, and usually helpful. Both instances reveal two scenarios which are not easy to come by – Rupali was in the US at the time she reports in the above dialogue, whereas Jitendra's "treatment" is handled by a cousin. The opportunity for counselling that Rupali had access to, and having a counsellor who was not medicine-oriented are opportunities few get. Jitendra's situation of having a cousin who supported him is also an unlikely situation for the vast number of people. Yet in one way or another, both Rupali and Jitendra were supported in looking beyond diagnostic labels. His cousin helps Jitendra to taper off medication after taking them for nearly six years, whereas Rupali eventually switches over to homeopathy.

Agency, responsibility, maintaining continuity

Any action is brought about by an agent who initiates and carries it through. In "psychosis" too, someone takes responsibility for decisions and their outcomes. It may be logical to believe the one experiencing a "psychosis" or meltdown would be momentarily unable to discern the right course of action, for the reality of those episodes is far removed from the daily reality of other's lives. In this book, the narrative of Akshay is an exemplar of such differences.

> *I had a sudden urge to turn inward … I broke many things in my room that night. I had made a (symbolic) "dead body" of flutes representing a head, and there was a flute for the heart, also broken. I pissed around the room and it all felt as though part of a ritual. Then when my father came, he gave me* paranthas *to eat. I threw them on the "dead body". I thought they would understand it all.*

he says

These words testify his experience or its perceived reality completely alien from others'. It made little sense to his father, who in his affection gave him something to eat his mother had lovingly sent. But Akshay was not in any frame to understand such love at the time. He was gripped by his own sense of "reality" trying to convey in it the symbolic realm, hoping someone else would comprehend. He admits *turning inward* as though attempting withdrawal from a world which had wounded him. He symbolically represents his wounding by a "dead body" he creates. In his symbolism, there seems to hide a metaphor of broken communication or music – as broken flutes. Yet his metaphors are not received in the manner they are expressed, for nobody understands the story in his mind. I see this as broken communication and entry into a domain where the symbolic dimension takes over what those around see real. The communication intended cannot be deciphered by anyone who cannot decode the symbolism. Dotson (2011:238) signifies the necessity of "being heard" as a point of speaker-dependence on audiences. Every speaker needs certain kinds of reciprocity for successful linguistic exchanges. Speakers are vulnerable in linguistic exchanges because an audience may or may not meet the linguistic needs of a given speaker in a given exchange. In the preceding exchange, the son's communication is not recognized by the father, making the former's actions incomprehensible and absurd to the latter. That Akshay is not heard for what he is conveying but literally for the spectacle that meets the eye creates an exchange which may be seen as nonsensical from the father's perspective. Naturally enough such communication fails for both son and father.

For any person seeing their loved one in a situation as Akshay's, to look for a psychiatric solution may appear rational, as it did his father and brother-in-law. The psychiatric option was duly explored, prescription sought and taken, and they chose to bring him home from university at least for a few days. But when he decided to return back after those few days, nobody insisted he should stay.

> *After I reached home, my whole family gathered around. I had discussions with them. I was practicing yoga ... I was into great disciplines. They made me stay for two days, and I convinced them to let me go. And they did. I went back to my university, stayed by myself. My friends and girlfriend would force me to take medicines. I had a fight with them, and they let me be. By such time I was singing "bhajans" having a "happy time". But I had to go home like everyone later. Throughout this period I was making my art. Then I was home for two months, the "highs" passed away and I became calmer. There were times I could not sleep, two-three days at a time.*

Even though Akshay returned home without resistance that they never forced him to stay back beyond a short time is a telling comment on the two sets of people. Not only was he coherent enough to assert his independence, they were also accommodating enough to (a) not force medication and (b) let him express his independence by going back. Paradoxically, upon return to the university, the insistence on medication he had overcome in this family came back from his friends, who had lesser opposition to psychiatry than him. It seems quite remarkable in the constant and continued negotiation for/against psychiatric medication he anyhow held his ground. He neither relented, give up his opposition to medication, nor let anyone have their way with him. No matter what his suffering, he refused to accept a label for it and made constant efforts to deal with it the best manner he could.

Who plays the major role in a person's life and decision-making process about issues concerning them, determines agency. Is someone themselves taking their own decisions or is someone else taking them on their behalf? Independent or dependent, autonomous or aided, self or other-driven, these distinguishers determine how people respond to most aspects of their life. It also impacts ideas about illness, pathology, career choices, marriage or partnerships, and scores of other dimensions in someone's life. In certain cases, someone may straightaway opt-out of psychiatric medication. If not coerced by families, they may continue finding their self-expression, and in time work a way out of suffering that works best for them, without constant supervision.

Citing research, Dressler et al. (2019:2) note there is no reason individuals cannot harness their own sense of self-efficacy and control in the world to pursue culturally constructed goals. Akshay harnesses his ability to gain control over his life, rather than concede to professionals determining the course of his distress. This is what may be seen as agency or "an individual's socio-culturally mediated capacity to act" (Ahearn, 2000:112). Ortner (2006) gives an exposition of the meaning of agency as a process which has a series of components. These components are (a) intentionality, (b) cultural and historical construction, and (c) its relationship with power. Even though agency is seen to be a universal phenomenon (e.g., see Sewell, 1992), and all humans have a capacity for agency, but the specific forms it takes will vary in different times and places (Ortner, 2006:136). Ahearn (2000:113) believes it is important to ask how people themselves conceive of their own actions and whether they attribute responsibility for events to individuals, to fate, to deities or to other animate or inanimate forces. These peers after understanding their "patient" status still keep taking decisions, moving onward with their lives instead of seeking constant professional or parental validation. They exhibit certain autonomy from the beginning.

Rupali decided to search for homeopathic solutions on her own, as she was looking for a way out of psychiatric medication. While her in-laws or husband did not contribute in this process she did not wait for them either. Though her natal family supported her choices, her own insistence on seeking alternatives was also nothing short of tenacious. She went from doctor to doctor, clinic to clinic alone sitting in queues everywhere in the hope *the right thing* was somewhere to be found.

> *Search for alternatives was a significant and persistent search. I kept looking one after the other. I went to one homeopathy institute, and sat waiting for six hours hoping they would be able to help me. But they also had some young people who were handing out prescriptions and it produced no difference from whatever they recommended to me.*
>
> – Rupali

She did not quit searching which seems quite incredible. Her faith in alternative (medical) systems never made her surrender to psychiatric ideas. Considering she had another "patient" as sibling her insistent search may appear contrary to expectation or, in fact, the reverse: propelled to search for an alternative for both, having seen the outcomes in one life closely.

Family's assistance towards recovery

There is a difference in the role played by families in instances where recovery occurs. While all parents exhibit an identical response in seeking psychiatric intervention, there was something additional in case of the parents of these three individuals[2] – *respecting the autonomy of the person*. This catalytic role facilitates expression of individual agency and assists "patients" in their quests. These families did not pose impediments due to their own learned or pre-existing ideas, biases or proclivities for choosing certain treatments over others. In fact, none insisted upon adherence to psychiatric regimens. They supported their children find their expressions and respected choices they made: whether Rupali switching to homeopathy, Jitendra tapering off psychiatric medication with the cousin's support or no insistence on psychiatric medication as visible in Akshay's story. It is not as if these families experienced lesser trouble themselves or Rupali's, Jitendra's or Akshay's behaviours were any less disturbed, socially "inappropriate" or "dysfunctional" than other peers'. But their respective parents' responses made a significant difference than if they had insisted on either taking psychiatric approval for stopping medication,[3] or disallowed them to look for other alternatives.

Narrative reconstructions

No doubt agency is an important determinant of recovery, but merely taking agency in treatment related decisions may not be enough for someone to recover. For people to move their stories outside the professional purview involves a profound assumption of personal responsibility (Frank, 1997:13). Several kinds of efforts are required to bring order out of the chaos, to bring life back on its rails, further from where derailment occurred. After stopping medicine, it may be time to meet other goals of life like another person, join broken pieces which can be mended, set and meet age appropriate milestones.

A common thread in each recovery narrative is treating distress as a phase, not letting it become an entire life. Though their on-going schedules was jeopardized, these individuals ensured the phase did not dominate their life. Each returned and completed unfinished tasks, not leaving midway, no matter how intractable. Rupali earned her Ph.D., Jitendra completed his bachelor's and Akshay took his master's degrees, in their respective universities. Each embraced the challenge of rejecting a discourse based on personal deficits and illness categories and created a new narrative.

---

2 Sona's mother also had an identical attitude, but given Sona's insistence on psychiatric medication she did not argue with her on the subject and let her have her way.

3 Many caregivers in this study insist on it and remain insistent even if their children wish to stop medication.

Gergen (1997:195) distinguishes forms of self-narratives in social life, into three rudimentary templates. These are the stability narrative, progressive narrative and the regressive narrative.

> The *stability narrative* depicts a case where the events of a person's life remain essentially unchanged in relation to a goal or an outcome. *Progressive narrative* links together events so that the movement along the evaluative dimension over time is incremental, and the *regressive narrative*, in which the movement is decremental.
>
> (ibid.)

All forms of self-narratives enumerated by Gergen are visible among the narratives of this study. Those who remain "patients" have a *stability narrative* remaining "patients". Whatever else they do, the underlying thought of their "patienthood" remains intact. So does a belief in and acceptance of the "patient" identity. Many among them actively seek ways towards recovery, being on medication, for the "patient's" role has not completely debilitated them, it is but one aspect of their lives. A majority of peers belong to this group.

HETAL: *"I see myself as ... like it's okay, it will work out. It's not the way I felt earlier for I would be quite worried. But now it doesn't bother so much. It is just okay".*
ME: *"So what is the reason for not worrying now?"*
HETAL: *"Now, it's just that I have things which occupy my mind, so I don't have time to worry".*

Having tried feasible alternatives since nothing seemed to offer certainty or a viable long-term alternative, they continue taking medication. This is also the sub-group that quizzed me minutely on many aspects of my recovery and compared notes with me over time, even though my research interviews with them were a one meeting affair. There is another group wherein decades of medication have made "patients" and families resign to the "patient" role; they do not seek a way out, having exhausted all visible options. As co-morbid conditions start appearing in time, partially also iatrogenic, their narratives turn *regressive narratives*. The difference between these two sub-groups, both taking medication, is while the latter does not seek alternatives, the former is still hopeful, open to new ideas, solutions and possibilities.

> *Nowadays if I go out also I am worried, if other people will find out that I am schizo ... aaa ... a schizophrenic patient, because I am just forgetting everything now and so I am getting afraid to talk to others also.*
>
> – Vindhya

141

Even though Vindhya does not take much medication[4] but a span of three decades of medication has created a deeply entrenched helplessness.

VINDHYA: *"I am afraid that people will know that I am schizophrenic. Like that I am afraid".*
ME: *"Even if they find out what can they do?"*
VINDHYA: *"No ma'am I will not find a job ma'am, till the end I will not find a job".*
ME: *"Till the end of what?"*
VINDHYA: *"Till the time I am good physically ma'am".*

The regressive narrative appears in those narratives where people not only remain on psychiatric medication but accept the sick role in all seriousness, progressively becoming weaker. Vindhya herself takes a dark, pessimistic view of her situations all the time. Even though a lot can be salvaged, her attitude itself ensures a downward slide. Living amidst fears of being discovered "schizophrenic" or belief that she cannot hold a job appear as self-fulfilling prophecies not permitting her to heal, without her realizing how close she may be to recovery. No matter how many times I have tried sharing with her how strong she is that she manages to live alone, conduct her daily affairs in spite of challenges, it is the negative self-construal that dominates our dialogue over the years.

The recovery narrative, on the other hand, is a progressive narrative. Even when people accept psychiatric medication, while not specifically targeting recovery, they still try to deal with their distress more actively rather than surrendering to the diagnosis. Given an option and no insistence on compliance from families they opt out of psychiatry the moment an opportunity appears. Or, they even quit without an alternative for they are convinced they do not gain from the medicine. In a *progressive narrative*, not only agency but a sense of self responsibility is equally noticeable. Rupali, Jitendra and Akshay are testimony what it takes to construct a progressive narrative notwithstanding facilitation from the milieu.

Dealing with stigma

The stigma of "mental illness" impacts people in crippling ways proving an obstacle in rehabilitation and recovery. At times in the midst of a "psychotic" moment or phase, the person may act out in pronounced, public ways, involving many around them, inviting unnecessary attention. But when the "psychotic" flares subside, they still have to go back

4 In fact she informed me she only took one medicine to help her sleep and nothing else, at the time I interviewed her.

into the same milieus and pick up their scattered pieces from the charred remains that linger. This return back into society can be scary. How does the individual and family deal with the *gaze* that may enter their lives during such episodes? Do they talk about their or their loved one's mental health issues with others to offer explanations? Seek support or join organizations to seek support from similar others who suffer?

JITENDRA: *"I did not have also any stigma as such actually ... but I was aware ... I did not have self-stigma. I started looking different that time I ... did not give (much emphasis) ... there was lesser knowledge about the severity of schizophrenia, nobody knew so much".*
ME: *"Did your family ever share with others outside the family, say relatives or neighbours, about your diagnosis?"*
JITENDRA: *"No, I don't think so".*
ME: *"You don't think so?"*
JITENDRA: *"Only ... very close people, may be one or two sisters of my mother".*

Keeping a stigmatizing identity under close wraps appears to have its advantages. It seems to help if people are left alone when someone is suffering deeply, instead of facing quizzical or prying eyes; it reduces immense pressure on the suffering individual. It especially proves advantageous when the "patient" needs time to heal from a deep suffering that foments a "psychotic" episode. By keeping quiet families protect their loved ones from the stigma and loss of social capital that diagnosis may bring and jeopardize future prospects in diverse domains. I first witnessed this among parents whose children still take psychiatric medication, and later saw it confirmed in the narratives of those who recovered. Keeping diagnosis-related information guarded is usually better than talking about it publicly.

I have noted earlier when there was a need to support their children, the mothers of both Rupali and Akshay stayed with their respective children. Their companionship on university campuses offered their children presence, support and courage to face the ripples of what may have stirred during their "psychosis". Having a familiar, reliable person to fall back on during periods of intense uncertainty always proves helpful. Both Rupali and Akshay experienced episodes during their time at university, far from home. Having parents during those phases when they returned to university and tried rebuilding their lives appears timely. It also helped mitigate the stigma of having said or done things construed "unseemly".

Recovery is possible both with/out psychiatric assistance, the former if a psychiatrist can help with tapering-off medication, and continuous rehabilitation efforts of a "patient". It also depends upon other environmental factors and proximity to triggers. In this book *all* recoveries happened in the absence of psychiatry's formal support. Although Jitendra's cousin supports weaning off the medication, he himself made other rehabilitation efforts that assisted his eventual recovery. Jitendra's case is somewhat atypical for most can only refer back to their doctors, who are not supportive of tapering off medication. Therefore, his narrative may also be beyond psychiatric gaze, albeit having informal support of psychiatry.

Rupali and Akshay found their solutions by vehemently rejecting the psychiatric option: the former after a few years and the latter soon after diagnosis. Equally so having families willing to support such choices are also not easily heard of. It needs elaboration that it is not as though these people are denying distress or its "psychotic" manifestations. Each of them went to a psychiatrist and obtained a diagnosis, before deciding on further course. A complete denial of distress, brushing it out of view so it shows up in disturbed behaviours for life is not the case: only the psychiatric solution is rejected at a sufficiently empowered and coherent stage when the individual is able to exercise their *will and preference*;[5] exhibiting agency, taking responsibility. Either ways, all three narratives suggest people can recover and sustain recoveries. These are such testimonies.

---

5 The idea of *will and preference* is an important constituent of the next chapter which discusses legal choices available to people and whether they are able to access them.

6

MAKING THE TRANSIENT PERMANENT – HOW LAW IMPEDES RECOVERY

"Persons with disabilities all across the world have faced discriminatory treatment and egregious human rights violations on a daily basis. Now, finally, we have a solid international legal framework in place that should allow them to cast off restrictions that have been placed on them by the rest of society."

"The 50-article Convention fights discrimination in relation to a wide range of rights that are often not accorded to persons with disabilities, either deliberately or through neglect. These include the rights to education, health, work, adequate living conditions, freedom of movement, freedom from exploitation and equal recognition before the law."

Arbour (2008)

The miniscule evidence proffered in Chapter 5 suggests recovery is well-nigh possible in India, albeit beyond the psychiatric gaze. This evidence encourages us to consider an extant possibility: if people can recover using their own means, possibly they can recover with greater certainty in lesser time if meaningfully supported by professionals. Instead, the latter focus on funnelling more people into the formal mental health system firmly believing their self-propagated myth of "lack of psychiatric infrastructure" (Murthy, 2011, Mills & Hildberg, 2020), a claim according to which vast populations are either underserved or improperly serviced for mental health issues in India and, more generally, in the entire low and middle income countries (LMICs) globally. In spite of "treatment" claims, medical services are unable to assist a majority of individuals recover from their setbacks and distress. Many become progressively disabled by whatever is offered in the name of "treatments". Wherein lay the gaps, what goes wrong and what goes behind a never ending dependence on "treatments"?

In Chapter 5, I examined the differences between family attitudes where recoveries occur and where they don't. These are the first level micro barriers. I propose micro-barriers exist within relational matrices which are

DOI: 10.4324/9781003248804-8

simultaneously ensconced within the larger macro-environment. This, in turn, is constituted by institutional mechanisms which operate normatively, privilege certain knowledge claims, create media for their dissemination and implementation, and ensure perpetuity of "treatment" regimens no matter what changes are made by which legal or policy instrument.

How the macro-environment thwarts people's recovery efforts constitutes this chapter. Discourse analysis points towards three interrelated ideas: (a) everyone looks for a way to recover, and before coming to a psychiatric clinic people often seek other kinds of help, which ultimately directs them to seek psychiatric intervention, (b) a majority of "patients" seek alternatives over and above psychiatric "treatment",[1] (c) people who seek alternatives to psychiatry look for options without any/much guidance from their psychiatrists. While these ideas constitute the necessary conditions for recovery, they are not sufficient.

Therefore, I probe the macro-environment to unearth where the sufficiency criteria for recovery fall short, by not letting the necessary conditions consolidate into full-scale recoveries. The goal is to build on barriers present in individual narratives by now looking for their genesis in the macro-environment. I examine the macro-environment through the lens of recovery, and its impact on the micro-environment, even though on the face of it the former does not directly contribute either to "patienthood" or recovery.

This scrutiny is inaugurated by analysing the Convention for Rights of Persons with Disability[2] (CRPD, or Convention), a comprehensive human rights document created with phenomenal participation by people with disabilities, including users and survivors of psychiatry (Davar, 2014:270). Focus lies on those aspects of the Convention which are relevant to advancing recovery, by juxtaposing the conceptual recovery categories with

---

1 In this book Rupali switched to homeopathy, Jitendra mentioned about peer support, Aditya decided on doing art based and yogic practices, Sona tried Chinese medicine, Nithya took the path of *ayurveda*, Hetal went to the Balaji temple in Mehndipur (Rajasthan), Smita tried everything possible: staying at a psychiatric rehabilitation centre, peer support, counselling (principally with her psychiatrist), Bhavna mentioned homeopathy for other health issues though not for mental health. Overall a majority of peers except Vindhya, Bhavna & Bharati tried some alternative form of intervention or support apart from mainstream psychiatry.

2 The CRPD is a Human Rights Convention which has been negotiated by all States who are members of the United Nations. Once adopted by the General Assembly, the Convention was opened for signature. Signing the Convention means that the State has agreed to not do anything which is contrary to the Convention. Ratification means that States have agreed to be bound by the Convention. The ratification can be with or without reservation. When a State files a reservation, it is saying that it will not be bound by that part of the Convention. Ordinarily, a State cannot enter into a reservation which is against the object and purpose of the Convention. However, when is a reservation considered permissible and when not is a contentious question.

provisions of the Convention. It is not as though the Convention specifically targets recovery as a goal, but whatever provisions it creates in supporting people's agency or capacity to emerge and their treatment/healing choices to be broadened constitute affirmative measures as far as the individual "patient" is concerned.

Thereafter I analyse the Indian Mental Healthcare Act 2017 (MHCA) and the mental health policy (MHP) in the light of the Convention to determine the extent to which the statutes advance the goals promoted by the Convention.

The conceptual recovery categories that emerged in Chapter 5 from individual narratives are: (a) developing agential capacity, (b) discontinuing psychiatric medication, (c) rehabilitation efforts and (d) family's non-insistence on psychiatric compliance. In addition to the necessary conditions for recovery these are the additional sufficiency criteria. My submission is if these four-five[3] things occur for someone they would recover many aspects of their life; possibly exit the "patient" role. These enabling factors are *not* visible in the lives of a vast majority of "patients". So, here lies an opportunity to revisit these narratives to probe, since they are unable to develop their agency, give up psychiatric medication or fulfil any of the other requirements for recovery, what part of the social policy landscape becomes a deterrent?

From the point of view of a "patient", it is their *will and preference* which is of paramount importance in determining recovery, for is someone's wellness *not* subjective? It is this will and preference which makes people seek psychiatric treatment in the first place. Therefore upholding it ought to remain central to determining recovery. However, the individual seen competent and rational at the time of *seeking* "treatment" is deemed irrational or lacking testimonial viability upon receiving a diagnosis. From this ambivalence between determining a person in/competent upon diagnosis and acknowledging their capacity as a legal subject, capable of taking decisions, we begin this inquiry.

Macro-environment ensconcing micro-environment

The epistemic scaffolding of this chapter begins from this fork in the road: how the individual seeking "treatment" and becoming "patient", is given legitimacy by the Convention. Prior to the CRPD in every legal and policy instrument this legitimacy was denied. Two attributes in the macro-environment, which can become catalysts for recovery, whose

---

3 The fifth attribute is how a person deals with stigma. It is not a conceptual category that necessarily emerges from my findings but how a person and family deals with stigma determines how a person takes control over their life, by not internalizing stigma and isolating oneself socially, which happens in a large number of instances.

tangibility was predicated in the preceding chapters, are (a) a plurality of treatment or healing options and (b) recognition of legal capacity. If these two conditions are present in the macro-environment, over and above the necessary conditions in the micro-environment, recovery can materialize.

I analyse the Convention to see the manner it creates opportunities for recovery. Does it privilege the hitherto marginalized voice of the "patient" to speak for herself, choose "treatments" and accept or reject psychiatric options equally? How is the question of force addressed in the Convention, the MHCA and the MHP? My focus within the Convention is a twofold analysis: (a) what enabling conditions does it create for abetting recoveries, and (b) what in the Convention are Indian law and policy expected to conform with? While there may be several recommendations for harmonization of the MHCA with the Convention, my core investigation remains the sufficiency criteria for recovery. How each of these instruments – the Convention, MHCA and MHP, enable recovery is my principal concern.

I repeat myself when I say necessary conditions in the macro-environment, over and above the sufficient conditions in the micro-environment have to come together for viable, long term recoveries. It would be pertinent to affirm that two key ingredients, both in macro-environments, constitute the final axis for recovery. Since both conditions are present in the macro-environment they have a direct bearing on the micro-politics of mental health, consequently choices people can exercise.

These two criteria are *legal capacity* and *medical pluralism*. Both of these are outcomes of the macro-environment yet come into effect via the micro-environment in people's relationships. My goal now is to keep these as my focus and minutely comb through all policy instruments and analyse how legal capacity and medical pluralism are defined, acknowledged, denied or upheld. This forms the red-thread of this analysis, holding which I advance my investigations of the macro-environment of "mental health" in India.

The CRPD – breaking new ground on disabilities

UN High Commissioner for human rights Louise Arbour (2008) identified the CRPD as a "ground-breaking" catalyst for change, marking the paradigm shift from viewing persons with disabilities as objects of charity and medical treatment to identifying them as subjects with legal rights. The CRPD is the most up-to-date international legal instrument specifically tailored to stipulate the rights of persons with disabilities. Such persons are taken to include those with serious mental disorders (Szmukler, 2019:34). The Convention creates several provisions that bring persons with disabilities (PwD) at par with all citizens in society, in every country that has ratified the Convention.[4] In the "General Principles"[5] it lays down several guidelines which aim to restore the dignity of PwD, which was hitherto denied to such individuals.

Traditionally, law has viewed the person who is disabled with prejudice and judged her to be incompetent. From an examination of disability laws, Dhanda (2007) notes that across jurisdictions, PwD are attributed incompetence in a legal sense in three ways: (a) status attribution – once their status as a PwD is established it is presumed they lack the ability to perform certain kinds of legal tasks; (b) functional test – a PwD is considered incompetent if due to disability they are unable to perform a specified function; and (c) outcome test – by watching the manner in which a PwD arrives at a decision. In the last context, their decision-making capacity is especially suspect if they are given a "mental illness" diagnosis. The crux is until the Convention most laws were focused on proving the incompetence of someone disabled, construing disability to be a personal flaw and weakness. Consequently, the individual was adjudged legally "incapable" or "incompetent".

Article 4 of the CRPD[6] places certain "General Obligations" on State parties which have far-reaching consequences on individual rights and opportunities. From the point of view of achieving recovery, Section 1(b) of Article 4[7] appears to create the first meaningful scope for changing debilitating mechanisms, including abolition of discriminating laws and practices. Going further it also proposes[8] that if professionals working with PwD are not capable of supporting individuals their further training and skill enhancement should be done, so they can serve those requiring their services in better ways. For a "patient" or caregiver, perhaps nothing is as potentially affirmative as this provision, which delimits the scope of psy-professionals from merely recommending pharmacological solutions and encourages them to look for alternative ways to serve the people they are meant to.

---

4 CRPD, Article 1: The purpose of the present Convention is to promote, protect and ensure the full and equal enjoyment of all human rights and fundamental freedoms by all persons with disabilities, and to promote respect for their inherent dignity.

5 CRPD, Article 3: (a) Respect for inherent dignity, individual autonomy including the freedom to make one's own choices, and independence of persons; (e) Equality of opportunity. (a) and (e) are the two subsections of Section 3 that has relevance to this discussion.

6 CRPD, Article 4: States Parties undertake to ensure and promote the full realization of all human rights and fundamental freedoms for all persons with disabilities without discrimination of any kind on the basis of disability.

7 CRPD, Article 4, Section 1(b): To take all appropriate measures, including legislation, to modify or abolish existing laws, regulations, customs and practices that constitute discrimination against persons with disabilities.

8 CRPD, Article 4, Section 1(g): To promote the training of professionals and staff working with persons with disabilities in the rights recognized in the present Convention so as to better provide the assistance and services guaranteed by those rights.

Article 5 of the CRPD[9] discards prejudice against those formerly considered "incompetent", and establishes equality and non-discrimination as the basis of inclusion of PwD in society. It builds on this provision further in Article 8 and attends to awareness-raising.[10] From the perspective of "patients", this could be an empowering provision as it aids inclusion of people diagnosed "mentally ill" in day-to-day situations which ordinarily they shy away from, for it may assist their rehabilitation efforts considerably. Further into the Convention, Article 9 creates accessibility for the PwD at all levels.[11] Some of these seem especially meaningful for promoting recovery by making information accessible. "Patients" and caregivers[12] often do not know the goals of psychiatric "treatment" and/or whether alternatives exist, or where. Making such information available to people fosters access to extant options, by extension medical pluralism.

Article 12 – catalyst for change

Legal capacity is the ability to hold rights and duties (legal standing) and to exercise those rights and duties (legal agency). Legal capacity includes the capacity to be both a holder of rights and to be an actor under the law. Legal capacity to act under the law recognizes that a person is an agent with the power to engage in transactions and create, modify or end legal relationships.[13] It is the key to accessing meaningful participation in society.[14] In this context, Article 12[15] of the Convention is seen as the

9   CRPD, Article 5, Section 2: States Parties shall prohibit all discrimination on the basis of disability and guarantee to persons with disabilities equal and effective legal protection against discrimination on all grounds.
10 CRPD, Article 8, Section 1 (*b*) To combat stereotypes, prejudices and harmful practices relating to persons with disabilities, including those based on sex and age, in all areas of life;(*c*) To promote awareness of the capabilities and contributions of persons with disabilities.
11 In particular the provisions in Article 9, Section 2(*c*) To provide training for stakeholders on accessibility issues facing persons with disabilities; and 2(f) To promote other appropriate forms of assistance and support to persons with disabilities to ensure their access to information.
12 I propose that knowledge of treatment options is a human rights issue, and denial of such information amounts to injustice. Fricker (2013) extends the idea of epistemic injustice as capable of producing another form of injustice, which she refers to as *distributive epistemic injustice* – the unfair distribution of epistemic goods such as education or information. I propose that the lack of information about non-medical approaches amounts to distributive epistemic injustice.
13 General Comment 1. Article 12, Section 12 which notes the normative content of Art.12.
14 General Comment 1. Article 12, Section 13.
15 Article 12, CRPD: Equal recognition before the law. In the General comment to the CRPD, the Committee on the Rights for persons with disabilities notes that 'equality before the law is a basic general principle of human rights protection and is indispensable

most revolutionary contribution to the rights of PwD as it "did not just reaffirm all persons with disabilities as persons before the law; it also recognised their legal capacity in all aspects of life on an equal basis with others".[16] A leap, from being "incompetent" to having competence to express their will and preference, henceforth enjoying legal standing is seen as the most empowering opportunity created by the Convention. Naturally enough, it forecloses the option of forcible treatment or any form of coercion.

> Article 12 builds on existing international provisions to apply the right to equal recognition before the law to persons with disabilities. It comprises five paragraphs, and is modelled on the previous treaties to set out a right to legal capacity on an equal basis with others for persons with disabilities. The right to legal capacity it articulates encompasses both legal standing and legal agency.
>
> (de Bhailis and Flynn, 2017:7)

To foster agency,[17] the foremost condition is whatever form of help someone desires be respected: nothing imposed in their "best interest" or any which way. If they are unaware what kind of help could assist them, at least there could be a set of choices available to help them decide. But if every avenue for help only leads them down the path of biomedical "treatment", in what manner does it actually empower?[18] The idea of *will and preference* becomes meaningful in this context because it acknowledges that the person is capable of making decisions about herself and facing the consequences of her choices.

---

for the exercise of other human rights. The Universal Declaration of Human Rights and the International Covenant on Civil and Political Rights specifically guarantee the right to equality before the law. Article 12 of the Convention on the Rights of Persons with Disabilities further describes the content of this civil right and focuses on the areas in which people with disabilities have traditionally been denied the right. Article 12 does not set out additional rights for people with disabilities; it simply describes the specific elements that States parties are required to take into account to ensure the right to equality before the law for people with disabilities, on an equal basis with others. (CRPD/C/GC/1, 2014).

16 This was the second part of Article12, CRPD: States Parties shall recognize that persons with disabilities enjoy legal capacity on an equal basis with others in all aspects of life.

17 I have proposed in this research that agency is the first conceptual attribute for recovery to be actualized.

18 This not only includes the various medical choices, but all other psy-professionals also who more often than not end up funneling people into the mental health system, as their own ontological, epistemic and professional assumptions and goals are tied to it.

Five tenets[19] of Art.12 have been described by Quinn (in Arstein-Kerslake et al., 2017:406) as a "paradigm shift". They encourage legal systems to abandon the emphasis on identifying the point at which a person is unable to express their will and preferences and therefore unable to exercise legal capacity. Citing evidence, Arstein-Kerslake et al. (ibid.) note while some have argued that this shift is impractical, the CRPD committee has made it clear that legal capacity is an absolute, inviolable right: impairment "must never be grounds for denying legal capacity or any of the rights provided for in Article 12".

de Bhailis and Flynn (2017:9) note

> Article 12 paragraph 3 places an obligation on states to provide supports to enable persons with disabilities to exercise legal capacity. Paragraph 4 requires States Parties to create safeguards to ensure that persons with disabilities can exercise their legal capacity.

Having made these provisions and once all other observations[20] were published the focus shifted on how the law reform process might work in practice and toward the resulting domestic law-reform processes.

Art.12 has been hailed as by far the most important contribution to the rights of PwD, because without legal capacity all other rights can be invalidated. Legal capacity is the prime foundation that creates scope for recognizing other choices or decisions, the will and preferences legitimized. But without creation of a plurality of recovery options, even legal capacity becomes another rubber stamp.

Further provisions facilitating recovery in the convention

Many allocations in the Convention beyond the "Right to equal recognition before the law" can foster recovery. The scope created by Articles 4 & 5 is already mentioned above. Further contributions from Article 14,[21]

---

19 These are as follows: (a) equal recognition everywhere, before law, (b) legal capacity akin to others (c) provision of access to exercise legal capacity (d) safeguards to prevent abuse in accordance with international human rights law, (e) equal right to inherit property and financial affairs (CRPD, Article 12).

20 The principal among these was the General comment on Art.12 which clarified in detail how provisions of Article12 had to be interpreted by State parties.

21 CRPD, Article 14: States Parties shall ensure that persons with disabilities, on an equal basis with others. Section 1(b) (PwD) are not deprived of their liberty unlawfully or arbitrarily, and that any deprivation of liberty is in conformity with the law, and that the existence of a disability shall in no case justify a deprivation of liberty.

Article 19,[22] Article 21,[23] Article 23[24] and Article 24[25] can also reinforce certain aspects of recovery. Each of these either buttresses some aspect of rehabilitation, recovery, community integration or builds self-esteem. All may be seen as affirmative mechanisms capable of creating an empowering pathway, instead of repeatedly focusing on a disabling identity, or insisting on a particular way to "deal" with it.

Article 26[26] refers to the health needs of PwD and has a provision for continued training of professionals working in this field. This is of paramount importance instead of psy-professionals continuing with ineffective, debilitating and thereafter disabling "treatments" following a monolithic DSM-centred ontology. Article 27 creates provisions[27] supportive of recovery: principally employment, a cornerstone of rehabilitation. Everyone who can work could be given gainful employment, which augments their mental well-being by being within a space that does not treat them as "incompetent", requiring constant attention, "treatment" or care.

Taken together these legal provisions create several kinds of recovery support mechanisms, having positive outcomes for both "patients" and caregivers, creating scope so more may explore the goal of recovery. The best aspect of these provisions taken together is that the onus does not lie either on the individual, their family or even their doctor (micro-environment), but is shared more generally by society. In a diffused manner, people can come together to support someone, without particularly emphasizing on their mental health or stigmatizing them.

22 CRPD, Article 19, Subsection (b) Persons with disabilities have access to a range of in-home, residential and other community support services, including personal assistance necessary to support living and inclusion in the community, and to prevent isolation or segregation from the community; (c) Community services and facilities for the general population are available on an equal basis to persons with disabilities and are responsive to their needs.

23 CRPD, Article 21: Freedom of expression and opinion, and access to information.

24 CRPD, Article 23 (b): The right of all persons with disabilities who are of marriageable age to marry and to found a family on the basis of free and full consent of the intending spouses is recognized.

25 CRPD, Article 24: Education. In particular Subsections (c) and (d) are noteworthy. Subsection (c) Reasonable accommodation of the individual's requirements is provided; (d) Persons with disabilities receive the support required, within the general education system, to facilitate their effective education.

26 CRPD, Article 26, Section 2(b): States Parties shall promote the development of initial and continuing training for professionals and staff working in habilitation and rehabilitation services.

27 CRPD, Article 27, Section 1(a) Prohibit discrimination on the basis of disability with regard to all matters concerning all forms of employment, including conditions of recruitment, hiring and employment, continuance of employment, career advancement and safe and healthy working conditions;

The point to focus hereafter would be how individual countries respond to these provisions and their legal instruments change, how they implement these ideas and to what extent they move in the directions proposed by the Convention. Seen from my perspective clearly the Convention has created enough scope for people to recover. It has created diverse sets of rights, opportunities, and possibilities that are meaningful, favourable and inclusive at local governmental levels. This also brings me to the next curve on this road, towards the Indian Mental Healthcare Act 2017 and how many recommendations of the CRPD's have been incorporated in it, or how far it fosters recovery.

MHCA: "progressive" or wolf in sheep's clothing?

The MHCA 2017 states its objective[28] about provision of services for the persons with "mental illness" and that "it is necessary to align and harmonize the existing laws with the said Convention". This segment investigates the MHCA in two ways. I start by analysing its goals: whether/how it is a break from the past or more of the same, how the CRPD necessitates changes and how they are implemented in the act. First, I analyse the ontological, and justice frameworks based on which the MHCA is created. Second, I look at all the "new" and "progressive" provisions, minutely dissecting each to tease out whether new additions really empower or merely create an ideational phantasmagoria.

The MHCA received the nod of the Indian President in April 2017 and became operational law from July 2018 when it came into force. As compared to the earlier legislation, there were many changes in this legislation because India was obliged to align it with the CRPD. Whether or not these changes can support someone's recovery is the moot question. The various kinds of narratives analysed in Chapters 4 and 5 of this book constitute the central hub which guides me to discern what can or not support recovery for diverse people, in different settings.

At first glance the overarching assumption on which the MHCA rests stands clear: "mental illness" is an actual category of "disease" or "illness", having a biochemical basis requiring medical treatment. This ontological assumption is a polar opposite from the position which informs this book. Therefore, let us start from why ontological assumptions matter.

---

28 "An Act to provide for mental healthcare and services for persons with mental illness and to protect, promote and fulfil the rights of such persons during delivery of mental healthcare and services and for matters connected therewith or incidental thereto". Available at: https://prsindia.org/files/bills_acts/acts_parliament/2017/the-mental-healthcare-act,-2017.pdf on 26th February 2022.

"Mental illness" as permanent[29] versus transient: implications

Ontological assumptions create ecosystems which justify their bases. Historically "mental illness" has been considered permanent. Accordingly "treatments" have been based on a "disease management model", rather than a recovery[30] orientation. Recovery[31] is not mentioned in the MHCA as a goal at all, making the exercise privilege psychiatric ontology. The MHCA is anchored in the historical attitude towards psychiatric "illness" and has made provisions accordingly. Some assumptions behind the MHCA are (a) permanence of "mental illness", (b) lifelong treatment of "patients" using psychiatric medication, (c) need for greater psychiatric infrastructure.

The MHCA rests on an assumption that greater access to services ensures ethical, enabling and humane treatments, as well as inclusion of hitherto underserved populations (a frequent rhetoric of the Global Mental Health (GMH) Movement) into a servable social group. Its notable objective is to increase psychiatric infrastructure by increasing the number of psychiatrists and other psy-professionals per unit population, who further echo psychiatric knowledge and work professionally to fortify a colonial ontology. Citing Patel et al. Mills (2014:34) notes that GMH advocacy sets "mental illness" firmly within a public, global health agenda, advocating for ensuring inclusion of mental health on the global public-health policy agenda, and the effective integration of mental health care into every level of general health care. In response to the GMH advocacy, the Act explicitly mandates a multi-layered structure of bureaucratic machinery to implement the MHCA including formation of a Central Mental Health Authority[32] (CMHA), to be followed by State Mental Health Authorities[33] and further Mental Health Review Boards.[34] Each of these organizations has complex, hierarchical structures, and in each people with lived experiences are represented. While the latter have a nominal presence (one or two), others playing "professionals" roles (bureaucrats, psychiatrists or other

---

29 All mental health legislations in India starting from the earliest in 1858, until the latest in 2017 are based on the same assumption, so there is continuity in epistemic foundations and not much difference from the past in the current legislation as well.

30 Whenever I mention the term "recovery" I mean a *drug free personal recovery*, the way a patient would consider themselves "recovered" and not a medication-dependent "recovery" as suggested by psychiatrists.

31 This was not the case when the Ministry of Health and Family Welfare (MoHFW) made the following observation years before the MHCA was promulgated: "[P]ersons with mental illness should be treated like other persons with health problems and the environment around them should be made conducive to facilitate recovery, rehabilitation and full participation in society" (MoHFW, 2013:56).

32 MHCA 2017, Section 33–44.

33 MHCA 2017, Section 45–56.

34 MHCA 2017, Section 73–84.

psy-professionals) have bigger representation.[35] The Indian State seems to have thrown in its full power, replete with human, material and resource possibilities to ensure that the individual who needs "treatment" should be treated by fair means or foul, regardless professionals manage restoring their mental health. It is difficult to imagine how a top-heavy structure of this nature can ever facilitate individual recoveries when principally its goal is to create a governance machinery and get it going. More so without establishing toward what outcomes these efforts be directed.

Mental health concerns everyone; it is not the exclusive preserve of health professionals and health services, especially psychiatrists. Many other areas of society need a better input than a normative field trying to define human behaviour, which is often determined by a mix of economic, social, cultural, political, gender and scores of other intersectional issues. In India, caste, class and poverty also become significant contributors, and all these factors also need an acknowledgement in determining someone's mental health. One cannot simplistically evaluate people's mental health shorn of context. These actions are vital, alongside treatment and prevention of mental illness, for improved population mental health, and hence social and economic development in countries (Herrman and Swartz, 2007). To leave mental health status judgements or decisions to psy-professionals, whose professional interests are tied to it, may not be the best option for society as a whole. Would they not end up perpetuating diagnosis, or "treatment" more than healing or recovery?

---

35 For example, this is how a State Mental Health authority is to be constituted – (*a*) Secretary or Principal Secretary in the Department of Health of State Government – chairperson *ex officio*; (*b*) Joint Secretary in the Department of Health of the State Government, in charge of mental health – member *ex officio*; (*c*) Director of Health Services or Medical Education – member *ex officio*; (*d*) Joint Secretary in the Department of Social Welfare of the State Government – member *ex officio*; (*e*) such other *ex officio* representatives from the relevant State Government Ministries or Departments; (*f*) Head of any of the Mental Hospitals in the State or Head of Department of Psychiatry at any Government Medical College, to be nominated by the State Government – member; (*g*) one eminent psychiatrist from the State not in Government service to be nominated by the State Government – member; (*h*) one mental health professional as defined in item (*iii*) of clause (*q*) of Sub-section (*1*) of Section 2 having at least 15 years' experience in the field, to be nominated by the State Government – member; (*i*) one psychiatric social worker having at least 15 years' experience in the field, to be nominated by the State Government – member; (*j*) one clinical psychologist having at least 15 years' experience in the field, to be nominated by the State Government – member; (*k*) one mental health nurse having at least 15 years' experience in the field of mental health, to be nominated by the State Government – member; two persons representing persons who have or have had mental illness, to be nominated by the State Government – member; (*m*) two persons representing care-givers of persons with mental illness or organizations representing care-givers, to be nominated by the State Government – members; (*n*) two persons representing non-governmental organizations which provide services to persons with mental illness, to be nominated by the State Government – members.

The arguable point is can ideas *not* oriented towards recovery, resting on the assumption of permanence of "illness" create recovery outcomes? A "disease management" approach is likely to have different priorities from a "recovery-focused approach". The existing social ecosystem funnels people into the psychiatric system, through a diffused network of referrals. It all works in a centripetal manner and remains unidirectional. It does not accommodate "patient" subjectivities who may want to seek out a folk healer, a peer or some other service not offered by psychiatrists. At present, it robs people of their agency and pushes everyone towards a uniform, mostly biomedical "treatment" orientation. This is where the state really needs to step in and stop the pharmageddon (Healy, 2012) of psychiatry subsume every individual's quest for healing. After all, it may be expected of the state to keep a balance between individual autonomy and state paternalism (Dhanda, 2019:374).

Since the undergirding assumption of the MHCA is permanence and acceptance of "illness" as truth, to even view any further provisions of the legislation seems an exercise in futility. As I said at the start of this part, an ontological approach creates an ecosystem to sustain itself. An ecosystem is likely to be replete with professionals, services, belief and ideas which keep the system in place, maintain status quo. If any system is constructed on the idea of people's one-sided entry into it, the approach followed in the system would be markedly different than a system design wherein it is assumed that whoever enters will exit the system and needs support until they do. An entry-only system would have markedly different goals than a free flowing system where people can enter and exit at will.

To create the latter a different set of professionals, knowledge, beliefs and bases would have to be established. Whatever the status quoist system preserves will have to be weeded out. The CRPD has created enough scope for the emergence of a truly empowering "patient"-centric system and this book rests on the view what psy-professionals refer to as "mental illness" are transient states of distress; they needn't be treated as anything but. The MHCA rests on an opposite belief in surrendering its reason to psychiatric ontology based on permanence of "illness". This raises the question again, whether there is still any point in examining the existing system, whilst such a gaping split is visible so early into the scrutiny.

Yet, since the goal was not to examine MHCA's ontological assumptions but also the manner it attempts harmonizing Indian legislation with the CRPD, I investigate the new provisions which this legislation creates and whether they are genuinely "patient"-centric. I do not stop there but further examine the MHCA from a "patient's" perspective. I am curious to understand whether the conjecture that law is a meta-barrier to recovery is mere speculation or does it have a grain of truth?

For recovery, the twin options of *medical plurality* and respecting the *will and preferences* of the "patient" create the environment for people's agency to surface. If individuals only have a psychiatric option which they cannot reject, or choose something more conducive this discussion, whether law creates scope for recovery itself becomes redundant.

Bearing this, the focus now is those provisions which are said to advance the rights of "patients" and/or their legal capacity. While there is little doubt the MHCA is somewhat different from the earlier legislations, there is no fundamental change at a philosophical level, as I have elucidated earlier. While some changes have been made, possibly due to international accountability and honouring India's commitment to the Convention, whether they advance recovery will be soon clear.

Legitimizing medical plurality – a progressive measure

While studying the effects of medical plurality in South India Halliburton (2004) notes that outcomes in "developing" countries were seen to be markedly different from those in the "developed" parts of the globe, according to WHO studies. He studied the impacts of *ayurveda*, mainstream psychiatric treatment and religious healing in Kerala to suggest these outcomes. He proposes that having a number of therapies to choose from makes it more likely that a person will find a treatment that "fits" – that is, one that works for him or her because it meets the personality, desires or concerns of the patient (Halliburton, 2004:81–82). Possibly in keeping with this sensibility the MHCA creates an alternative potential for the "patients", via provisions for greater (treatment) options to choose from. As compared to the Mental Health Act of 1987,[36] which only allowed for homeopathic practitioners to offer mental health services, the MHCA creates further plurality, including *ayurveda, unani, siddha* and homeopathy.[37] However it tries to standardize their treatment procedures on the same lines as allopathy, which amounts to subsuming their epistemological basis under biomedicine's wingspan.

In the allopathic system, standalone medical establishments may work in mental health. Other systems of medicine *do not* have dedicated facilities devoted exclusively to mental health for they are often not based on a mind-body dualism. This creates a challenge how to make them part of a psychiatric

36 MHA, 1987, Section 2, clause (k) "medical practitioner" means a person who possesses a recognised medical qualification as defined, sub clause (iii) in clause (g) of Sub-section (1) of Section 2 of the Homoeopathy Central Council Act, 1973 (59 of 1973), and whose name has been entered in a State Register of Homoeopathy, as defined in clause (i) of Sub-section (1) of that section.
37 MHCA, Section 18, Subsection (10): Provided that where the health professional of ayurveda, yoga, unani, siddha, homoeopathy or naturopathy systems recognised by the Central Government are available in any health establishment, the essential medicines from any similar list relating to the appropriate ayurveda, yoga, unani, siddha, homoeopathy or naturopathy systems shall also be made available free of cost to all persons with mental illness.

establishment, and what becomes of their status. Do they operate as independent systems or adjuncts to psychiatry?[38] It is by hit and trial "patients" chance upon a solution that works for them, by often trying multiple options. So, though the presence of alternatives creates a potential for recovery and "patient"-centred environments, the salience of psychiatry diminishes all systems systematically. Summarizing, while policy creates scope for medical pluralism due to its normative psychiatry-led operationalization, all options other than psychiatry are either belittled, become invisible or made irrelevant.

Does the MHCA create options for recovery? Only closer scrutiny of the law can shed light on this. In what manner does the MHCA support the average[39] psychiatric patients, considering its claim of a "big leap from the 1987 act" (Kumar, 2018:106). There are many elements in the MHCA as response to the CRPD. Who do these new instruments end up supporting – "patients", caregivers or psychiatrists? As one of the key criteria for recovery – having a diverse set of "treatment"/healing options or medical pluralism is now mandated by the MHCA how will the *will and preference* of the patient, the other catalytic condition for recovery accommodated? This forms my next inquest.

MHCA: creating rights for what?

The chief purpose of a rights-based approach is to ensure that every person be given all rights enjoyed by another without discrimination based on any ground which segregates them from another such as religion, class, ethnicity, language, gender, nationality, caste, age or disability – transient or permanent. In this context Puras and Gooding (2019:42) suggest for psychiatrists and all healing professions, a pivot toward human rights would require setting aside "substitute decision-making" and offering support according to a person's "will and preferences", and where unknown, the "best interpretation" of her/his will and preferences.

Is this the manner the MHCA respects the rights of "patients"? Who defines *what* the rights are or ought to be? If anyone claims rights on behalf of "patients", what is the value of the claim of such a person/group? Does such a claim for another's rights have any conflict of interests in representing their own version of justice for another group? Is it tied to a professional position, does it have an ethical stance or is it shoring up the agenda of an invisible group and obliquely serving both interests? The latter is the pharmaceutical industry which has been widely censured for its treatment claims via the pharmaceutical options developed and marketed as a response to human distress, labelled "illness".

---

38 I have attempted to illustrate this by studying the working of a homeopathic center in Appendix D.

39 I consider myself an "average" psychiatric patient and the word is not implied in a pejorative sense.

Seen from a "patient" perspective when someone is temporarily dysfunctional, incoherent or disabled by "psychosis", they or their family may choose psychiatric intervention initially. But nobody wants treatment over decades. Choosing a treatment option ought not to mean they remain with it having no alternatives, which, in fact, happens routinely. Once treatments begin, they never seem to end! There are several aspects of the CRPD which offer insights on this issue.[40] These are cardinal issues from a recovery perspective. Otherwise being detained, forcibly treated, treated against their will, or disallowed from discontinuing treatment by in/formal coercion means people have "patienthood" imposed upon them: not allowed to exercise their rights of equality before the law or choose their "treatments". More crucially the Convention says should anyone decide to withdraw from medication *they should be assisted for it*, a significant move. A majority of "patients" would not wish to remain caught within the psychiatric web, yet people stay so for want of alternatives.

Let us briefly deliberate on the well-known phenomenon of coercion in psychiatry – which may be a uniquely disagreeable professional conduct – of imposing "treatments" on unwilling patients, a laurel shared by few medical specialties!

Psychiatric "treatment" and disability[41]

Before scrutinizing "treatments" and relevant MHCA's recommendations, I put forward the following idea: what is claimed "treatment" by

---

40 CRPD Guidelines on Article 14-23, adopted, Sep 2015. Section 24 subclause *d* and *e* of clause 126, by the Working group on arbitrary detention says "[i]ndividuals who are currently detained in a psychiatric hospital or similar institution and/or subjected to forced treatment, or who may be so detained or forcibly treated in the future, must be informed about ways in which they can effectively and promptly secure their release including injunctive relief".

> Such relief should consist of an order requiring the facility to release the person immediately and/or to immediately cease any forced treatment, as well as systemic measures such as requiring mental health facilities to unlock their doors and inform persons of their right to leave, and establishing a public authority to provide for access to housing, means of subsistence and other forms of economic and social support in order to facilitate deinstitutionalization and the right to live independently and be included in the community. Such assistance programs should not be centered on the provision of mental health services or treatment, but free or affordable community-based services, including alternatives that are free from medical diagnosis and interventions. Access to medications and assistance in withdrawing from medications should be made available for those who so decide.

41 To illustrate my point I have taken the case of Vindhya and attempted to explicate in what manner a person becomes patient, then progressively disabled. This illustration is developed in Appendix C by extracting from her narrative an excerpt relating to treatment and its outcomes. Taking her testimony as my base I researched for evidence from the literatures which pointed me towards co-morbidities and iatrogenic effects of psychiatric treatments to illustrate how long-term use of psychiatric medications debilitates.

professionals is not what "patients" necessarily want when they seek psychiatric help. But more importantly, continuing "treatments" over long spans of time, damage people.

> *I have the side effects. Due to tension my stomach gets upset often, probably more than once I go to release my stools. I discussed this with my doctor, he admitted it is a side effects of the antipsychotic drugs. He asked me to go to the physician related to the stomach, and told me that I have to live with it.*
>
> Vindhya

Vindhya developed several conditions due to her "treatment". How does one justify it and who takes responsibility? If we follow her life trajectory, the following is clear: (at the time of writing this) she is somewhat disabled by whatever side-effects have appeared in the long span (32+ years). Any scope for her to interact socially, take up a job, venture out of her home for a flexible amount of time, eating balanced meals has been fractured. She lacks courage, confidence and the supportive environment essential for recovery. Can she ever recover caught in the vicious, self-reinforcing grip of devastating beliefs?

When "treatments" continue, co-morbid conditions which are often side-effects of medications can push people towards greater instability, precarity, insecurity. More than a right to "treatments", it is a right to knowledge about "treatment" outcomes which seems more meaningful and "patient-centric". Vindhya is a typical chronic "patient"; never doubting psychiatric opinions. Her's is an unquestioning surrender to the psychiatric script, a helpless inability to express her actual suffering openly (e.g., the effect of medication on her bowels). Rimke (2018:16) proposes a critical framework of analysis which questions the way in which society makes women sick and then ultimately blames them for experiencing distress. She offers the idea of *psycho-centrism* as an oppressive practice in the same vein as the oppressive practices of neoliberalism, capitalism and other race, gender and identity based constructions.

> Psy-hegemony operates on different social levels and through multiple social mechanisms that blame the individual and thus erases the social context and social bases of women's distress and suffering. In neoliberalism, social problems have been reduced to individual pathologies, often embraced by the pathologized themselves.
>
> (ibid: 17)

Knowledge about "treatment" – a right of the patients

Either psychiatrists themselves do not know about (complete) recovery or they are aware yet believe it to be culturally irrelevant, for we do not have the public infrastructure necessary to support recovery. If recovery is not a goal of mental health treatment and services, then what is (Sharma, 2019a)? What scope does law offer to facilitate recovery? The MHCA states its objective: "to provide for mental healthcare and services for persons with mental illness and to protect, promote and fulfil the rights of such persons". Two things could be underscored: (a) mental illness construed as *real* illness, (b) foregrounding the rights of "patients". But once again who defines what those rights ought to be?

After all, mental health is not a monolithic truth without subjective individual variants. Someone may want to dance to feel good, another may want to go on a pilgrimage, discotheque or forest, someone may want to listen to pop music, another may write, do skating or go shopping! How does one nail down something so subjective? When definitions are so diverse, ambiguous, obscure what universal solutions can come for them? Even the same person may have different needs at different stages of life, or in different situations. It is not an objective phenomenon having material basis but a subjective reality of people, say for instance if someone feels afraid or angry. It can be supported with suitable other means from religion and faith in god/temples/ *dargahs* or any such spiritual activity, by engaging in art based activities: including expressive arts such as music, dance, theatre, plastic arts, writing and so forth. "The evaluation of wellbeing needs to be qualitative as well, as it requires an assessment of how the recipients feel about the programmes launched for their benefit" (Dhanda, 2019:374). Ruling out certain measures and insisting upon others stifles choices people may want in tune with their own sensibilities. Mental health is not created in isolation but from day-to-day experiences. Any setback can have a different outcome with different people, due to their different capacities for dealing with setbacks. Similarly the ability to recover from setbacks is a part of human responses. People suffer and reorganize their worlds all the time. Calling distress a diagnostic name is not helpful for recovery. Everyone understands what recovery means, they can extend the idea to their mental health equally.

If "patients" repose faith in psychiatrists, who never refer to recovery but warn[42] about worsening prognosis, would any "patient" have the capacity to heal or recover? In 32+ years of "treatment", Vindhya never heard from her psychiatrist that she was well enough to quit medication.[43] It may be clear from her story that "treatment" has disabled her, made her socially reclusive, diffident and perpetually anxious. The foremost rights people require are access to information about treatments. This information must be recognized as knowledge, rather than a right to information (RTI) query.

---

42 Does it not amount to informal coercion?
43 Even though she contacted me to discuss her "recovery" notwithstanding my testimony, for possibly she sees it as unreliable, she refuses to give up "treatment".

Fricker (2013:1318) suggests the lack of access to information may amount to distributive epistemic injustice.

We ought to legislate to create scope for dissemination of information about recovery, and ways to create more avenues to facilitate recovery. I still make the effort to examine the MHCA to scrutinize (a) where lays the scope for recovery in this statute, but more importantly (b) wherein lay those barriers which thwart recovery outcomes. The latter is pertinent as the ontological basis of "illness" creates structure geared towards "treating" people alone. Such assumptions are at odds with the belief mental distress is transient or it can be tidied over with less definitive "treatments".

MHCA and recovery

The ontological position underlying the MHCA being anchored in the "disease" model mandates infrastructural recommendations in consonance with it: more personnel, institutions, bureaucratic machinery and so on. I tease out each of these to exhibit how the growing edifice of infrastructure stymies any efforts of patients and families toward recovery, instead of assisting them heal. This legislation ensures that people remain within the lengthening shadows of gloom, progressively become disabled, visible in Vindhya's narrative. The goal is to see what would make her (or another) recover.

Definitional issues – mental health professionals and others

The MHCA has established medical plurality yet foisted allopathic norms on other systems of medicine, which do not operate on similar ontological principles. In particular, holistic systems such as homeopathy or *ayurveda* do not view the human body through the Descartian mind-body dualism. Their approach is systemic. But since the MHCA professionals trained in all systems of medicine can be designated "mental health professionals",[44] medical establishments[45] of all systems of medicine can be assigned a mental health establishment status. I exhibit the complexities of one such establishment by randomly selecting one homeopathy-based institution[46] to

---

44 MHCA, Section 2 (r): "Mental health professional" means a professional having a postgraduate degree (Ayurveda) in Mano Vigyan Avum Manas Roga or a post-graduate degree (Homoeopathy) in Psychiatry or a post-graduate degree (Unani) in Moalijat (Nafasiyatt) or a post-graduate degree (Siddha) in SirappuMaruthuvam.

45 MHCA, Section 2(p): "mental health establishment" means any health establishment, including Ayurveda, Yoga and Naturopathy, Unani, Siddha and Homoeopathy establishment.

46 Due to prior exposure from childhood I have a certain ease of comprehending homeopathy, therefore the choice of homeopathy, though the institution chosen is not known to me.

see the nature of work, research and services they offer in mental health (Appendix D).

Similarly, the Act has permitted postgraduates[47] with psychology degrees to be called "clinical psychologist". It conveys the underlying urgency to fill up vacancies in mental health anyhow and respond to the deficit in personnel (e.g., Kaur and Pathak, 2017, Kulkarni and Gaiha, 2017), the global mental health movement has been circulating since inception. Their training norms and criteria have been obfuscated and fudged to encourage more graduates into the mental health system, with low skills[48] to understand human mind by loosely matching people with DSM based classifications.

"Mental illness" and capacity to make decisions

Section 3[49] states how mental illness is to be defined. Interestingly though the next subsection[50] says people cannot be blamed in the present in case someone suffered from a "mental illness" in their past, it does not propose any measures or penalty in case someone does so.[51] When someone's past cannot be legally brought up for public scrutiny, if someone does so with the intention to malign them and prove them "incompetent" what intent does it reveal? Does it not evoke prejudice and stigma against the one vilified? Would not such a verbal violence impact anyone recovering from a mental health issue, without being public about their personal suffering? Why should the other person who spreads this information about another be allowed to go scot-free, without any penal outcome?

---

47 MHCA, Section 2(g): "clinical psychologist" means a person having a Post-Graduate degree in Psychology or Clinical Psychology or Applied Psychology and a Master of Philosophy in Clinical Psychology or Medical and Social Psychology obtained after completion of a full time course of two years which includes *supervised clinical training from any University* (emphasis supplied).

48 I have been a regular visitor and speaker in psychology departments around the country since 2007, where I meet post graduate students all the time. Though I find students inquisitive they are confused and troubled about classifications based on pathological categories. Yet their curricula often do not permit them the scope to look into other conceptualizations. They pass out of these degree programs with scant knowledge how to deal with mental health issues, having minimum exposure to analytical processes of understanding human distress. Most of their knowledge is normative and diagnosis-orientated.

49 MHCA, Section 3: Mental illness shall be determined in accordance with such nationally or internationally accepted medical standards.

50 MHCA, Section 3, Subsection (2): No person or authority shall classify a person as a person with mental illness, except for purposes directly relating to the treatment of the mental illness or in other matters.

51 In a recent case, in early 2019; of a well-known parliamentarian was found implicating someone in the public domain for their alleged history of mental health issues. The latter is a well-known and hails from a political family. Though it raised a hue and cry in the media for a few days there were no other outcomes (see Sharma, 2019a).

The next section[52] appears supportive of people's recoveries, if any person wants to take a decision about their mental healthcare treatment. However, I turn back to see whether someone really distressed is actually able to do it or what happens when they do not. I have discussed earlier (see Chapter 4) how everyone who looks for help is sooner than later referred to a psychiatrist, even if they may simply wanted to talk to someone to be relieved. A caregiver reflects,

Actually we didn't straightaway ... refer to a psychiatrist ... but a psychologist known to us, a friend. After one or two meetings that person referred us to a psychiatrist.

Bharati's mother

Even if the individual does not choose psychiatry, they are often guided towards it. In a majority of narratives, people in distress reach out to members of their respective families or close acquaintances seeking help. One or another way this cry for help further leads to psychiatry. I have exhibited repeatedly (Appendix B) how people are funnelled into the psychiatric system from diverse pathways. A law acknowledging people's capacity to seek out treatment seems a supportive law. Ironically, the law only leads people towards the psychiatric option – promising "treatments", without a cure!

It appears as though the capacity of an individual in their treatment related decisions is acknowledged, but there is no mention of the phrase *legal capacity*. That alone is the real measure which restores people's rights ensuring whatever decisions they make for themselves are respected when a need for implementing those decisions occurs: nobody treated in ways they do not wish. Overall this section does not seem to create clarity about how the capacity of a person or the *will and preferences* of the individual will emerge or given a scope to prevail.

Advance directive

Two provisions in the MHCA appear to respond to the above dilemma of *will and preference*. For its operationalization the MHCA creates two separate provisions: the first is the psychiatric advance directive (PAD) or simply advance directive (AD), and the second appointing a nominated representative (NR). The latter provision is also laid out in the AD as per this provision. In this subsection I focus on the AD and take up the NR in the next.

Campbell and Kisley (2009) define AD as a mandate that specifies a person's preferences for treatment, should s/he lose the capacity to make

52 MHCA, Section 4 (*1*): Every person, including a person with mental illness shall be deemed to have capacity to make decisions regarding his mental healthcare or treatment.

treatment decisions in future. Treatment choices, objections, values and principles can be stipulated in such documents. These directives first came to the fore in "end-of-life" care (Philip et al., 2019:S680). Before the UN-CRPD and the MHCA, "patients" could not have given valid advance instructions and expected them to be followed. One of the barriers would have been the presumption of *mental incapacity* that goes along with a diagnosis of mental illness.

The MHCA[53] gives the right to any person to give an advance directive in writing, via a complex, multi-stage process whose provisions include (a) the manner of making an advance directive in Section 6,[54] (b) maintenance of an online registry in Section 7, (c) revocation, amendment or cancellation of an AD, Section 8, (d) recommendation to not to apply AD to emergency treatment in Section 9, (e) duty to follow the AD and on whom it rests in Section 10 and (f) power to review, alter, modify or cancel AD in Section 11.

Even though the AD provision is created meticulously, in the next section,[55] the power to review the same has been created, which can more or less invalidate the AD. In other words, the implementation of the AD is not legally enforceable! So what is the *locus standi* of the AD? Is it just a piece of paper that the "patient" or future "patient" can hope would be followed, if their caregivers or psychiatrists are *kind enough* to accommodate their request? Yet the issue does not stop here, it goes further – until the Central Mental Health Authority[56] (also, Central Authority or CMHA), vested with the capacity to review AD. It is the next provisions[57] of Section 12, further problematic for recovery.

---

53 MHCA, Section 5: Every person, who is not a minor, shall have a right to make an advance directive in writing, specifying (*a*) the way the person wishes to be cared for and treated for a mental illness; (*b*) the way the person wishes not to be cared for and treated for a mental illness; (*c*) the individual or individuals, in order of precedence, he wants to appoint as his nominated representative.

54 MHCA, Section 6: An advance directive shall be made in the manner as may be specified by the regulations made by the Central Authority.

55 MHCA, Section 11 *(1)*: Where a mental health professional or a relative or a care-giver of a person desires *not to follow* (emphasis supplied) an advance directive while treating a person with mental illness, such mental health professional or the relative or the care-giver of the person shall make an application to the concerned Board to review, alter, modify or cancel the advance directive.

56 MHCA, Section 12 *(1)* The Central Authority shall regularly and periodically review the use of advance directives and make recommendations in respect thereof.

57 MHCA, Section 12, Subsection *(2)* The Central Authority in its review under Sub-section *(1)* shall give specific consideration to the procedure for making an advance directive and also examine whether the existing procedure protects the rights of persons with mental illness. Ibid, Subsection *(3)* The Central Authority may modify the procedure for making an advance directive or make additional regulations regarding the procedure for advance directive to protect the rights of persons with mental illness.

In both subsections, the phrase "the rights of the persons with mental illness" appears. As I have said again and again, the issue remains *who defines those rights*. When this legislation itself believes that it is the right of the persons to receive medical treatment, its view is predicated on the assumption that the medical treatment is *the* solution for the problem. Whether or not the medical treatment hurts (see Appendix C) is not recognized. A continued insistence on "treatment" circumventing the *will and preferences* of people by discarding their AD, whenever deemed necessary is a travesty of justice. Not only are the "patient's" rights dispensable, but their execution is also dependent upon the discretion of the macro-institutions of society, over and above family and psychiatry. If per chance someone overcomes barriers and looks for ways to recover, a paternalistic macro-environment may still insist on psychiatric compliance. This is what recognition of the "treatment" option as the rights of the "patient" amounts to.

This misgiving is confirmed by in the context of the "rights" of "patients" in Section 18 – wherein a long list of "rights" are listed. By-and-large, all of them lay within a psychiatric conception of what "rights" should look like, even though other medical systems are recognized here. In particular, Section 18, subsection (10) refers to a plurality of treatment options especially those of the AYUSH department. In this context, Cant's (2020:3) insight is noteworthy,

> Whilst plural healing modalities have (re)positioned themselves in the global marketplace ... biomedicine continues to shape the delivery and practice of health care, and to define what counts as legitimate knowledge. As such, medical pluralism has had limited impact on the epistemological and economic dominance of biomedicine which remains anchored by neoliberalism, capitalism and, importantly, the legacies of colonialism.

As confirmation, I have exhibited (Appendix D) how one alternative system – homeopathy, based on a different epistemological foundation reframes itself to match up with criteria established by psychiatry, operating as an adjunct, rather than asserting its own philosophical principles: "a premise that illness is a result of an imbalance of one's *vital force*, or essential energetic makeup. A correctly prescribed remedy leads to a restoration of the balance and ultimately to cure" (Merrell and Shalts, 2002:48).

Fricker's idea of epistemic justice to matters of political freedom appears befitting in this context. She likens this freedom to the relationship between a master and a slave wherein the freedom of the slave is a matter of discretion of the master. Transposing it on the relationship between psychiatry and "patients", the capacity of the latter becomes a matter of discretion of the former, no matter the advance directive.

> On this conception, real political freedom cannot be won through grace and favour, for grace and favour can only supply freedom de facto, and never freedom as of right. Mere de facto freedom, understood in terms of the relationship of ruler to ruled, is structurally speaking another species of tyranny, given that tyrants (like masters in general) need not be cruel but can be benign. The essentially tyrannical feature of the relationship here is the power relation that consists in the ruler's entitlement to rescind at will the freedoms bestowed upon the subject.
>
> (Fricker, 2013:1320–1321)

Continuing with the idea of coloniality of psychiatry (see Chapter 2), a critical analysis of law both confirms it and exhibits how legal functioning further entrenches coloniality. The present law can insist on the terms of the relationship even if both psychiatrist and/or "patient" refuse the terms! (Figure 6.1).

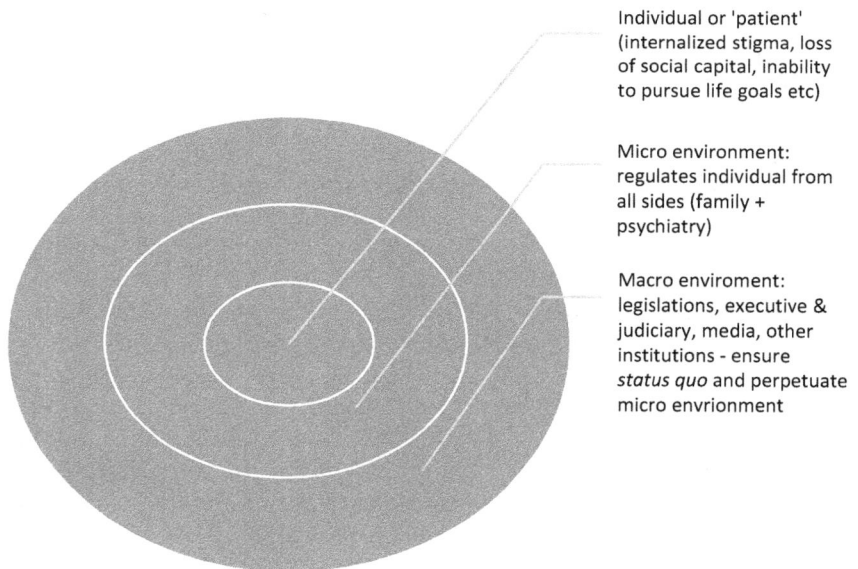

Individual or 'patient' (internalized stigma, loss of social capital, inability to pursue life goals etc)

Micro environment: regulates individual from all sides (family + psychiatry)

Macro enviroment: legislations, executive & judiciary, media, other institutions - ensure *status quo* and perpetuate micro envrionment

Figure 6.1 A conceptual representation of barriers to recovery depicted as three concentric circles nested within one another. The largest circle comprises the macro environment which contains the micro environment, which further sustains and keeps the individual "patient" in a stable "patient" role

To complicate matters the Central Authority[58] can also intervene: the state ends up directly intervening at the level of the individual to "ensure her rights"! This action appears to violate the legal capacity clause.

To illustrate: suppose someone has put an AD in place, the state has a right to modify the procedure or make additional regulations. But what happens to the AD once written – is it expected that the person would keep changing their AD every time the regulations change? Does it not appear as though the state is keeping the "patient" in its grip at all times? To revoke someone's preferred treatment by attributing "incompetency", or changing its provisions is a fallback on the same colonial mentality which has undergirded the history of mental health legislations in India. One is left to wonder in what manner the legal capacity of the "patient" is interpreted by the MHCA if this is how the AD works.

Not only from the "patient" perspective is an AD complicated and non-supportive psychiatrists also question the process of making such directives. "Section 81, stipulates that the central government is to create a guidance document for medical practitioners regarding capacity assessments. This will have an implication on PADs ... the MHRB has the powers to review, alter, or modify the PADs" (Philip et al., 2019:S682). This implies that ultimately the real power lies with the MHRBs, not even psychiatrists note Sarin et al. (2012:106).

Even though the MHCA creates a scope for advance directives, the process and its implementation are neither straightforward nor easy. The implementation and sustainability of the recommendations rests on environments conducive for the task. It becomes a foreclosed option when the AD can be challenged, questioned or revoked at every level. With an obstacle course set up does it really appear as if anyone is trying to support a "patient's" recovery? The multiple levels of in-built approvals makes it distasteful for anyone who requires such approvals, whether "patient", caregiver or psychiatrist.

Nominated representative

The advance directive can also be about a nominated representative[59] (NR): an individual responsible for taking treatment decisions during

---

58 MHCA, Section 12, Subsection (3): The Central Authority may modify the procedure for making an advance directive or make additional regulations regarding the procedure for advance directive to protect the rights of persons with mental illness.

59 MHCA, Section 5, Subsection (1), Every person, who is not a minor, shall have a right to make an advance directive in writing, specifying in clause (c): the individual or individuals, in order of precedence, he wants to appoint as his nominated representative.

periods of incompetence, should such a situation arise. The NR is defined in a comprehensive way and the person can be anyone from a non-minor relative[60] willing to discharge their duties under the Act, to a representative of the Department of Social Welfare,[61] who may act in the absence or unwillingness of a relative to take responsibility or anyone appointed with due authority by the Department. The Board is also vested with powers for revocation, alteration etcetera of the NR.[62]

Time and again the effort to empower everyone around the "patient" seems evident. This includes giving authority for making decisions for "patients" to any number of individuals who may be willing to discharge responsibilities as prescribed. Nowhere does one get a sense these provisions are made for someone who is considered competent to handle their issues, or as though their own capacity has legal sanction. Various checks and balances have been created within the system to ensure that given a little deviation, from the notional "normal" (which largely remains undefined or probably defined by the ICD[63] based classifications followed for this law) there would be clear cut ways to bring the person back into medical system.

The manner of AD creation, including its scope for nominating a person to represent the "patient", makes it an unlikely ally to advance the goal of recovery. To facilitate recovery the advance directive has to be completely, irrevocably *non-negotiable*. It ought not to require anyone else's approval for its implementation, nor overruled, redesigned or remodelled upon the discretion of any authority, including the MHRB. In the current format the advance directive invalidates most rights "patients" may have secured via

60 MHCA, Section 14 (3): The person appointed as the nominated representative shall not be a minor, be competent to discharge the duties or perform the functions assigned to him under this Act, and give his consent in writing to the mental health professional to discharge his duties and perform the functions assigned to him under this Act.

61 MHCA, Section 14: Where no nominated representative is appointed by a person under Sub-section (1), the following persons for the purposes of this Act in the order of precedence shall be deemed to be the nominated representative of a person with mental illness, namely Subsection (4e): if no such person is available to be appointed as a nominated representative, the Board shall appoint the Director, Department of Social Welfare, or his designated representative, as the nominated representative of the person with mental illness: Provided that a person representing an organization registered under the Societies Registration Act, 1860 or any other law for the time being in force, working for persons with mental illness, may temporarily be engaged by the mental health professional to discharge the duties of a nominated representative pending appointment of a nominated representative by the concerned Board.

62 MHCA, Section 16: The Board, on an application made to it by the person with mental illness, or by a relative of such person, or by the psychiatrist responsible for the care of such person, or by the medical officer in-charge of the mental health establishment where the individual is admitted or proposed to be admitted, may revoke, alter or modify the order made under clause (e) of Sub-section (4) of Section 14 or under Sub-section (2) of Section 15.

63 ICD refers to the international classification of diseases.

the CRPD, especially the choice of treatments, medical plurality and adherence to their preferred modes of support/treatment or healing.

Psychiatric "patient" at par with another

In the MHCA the issue of psychiatric medication is nested under "rights of persons with mental illness".[64] It appears an attempt to provide mental health services akin to other health services. The conceptualization makes it look like another physical health issue and implies mental health issues can be isolated in the body to be "fixed" when dysfunctional, like another part of the body. Here the normative assumption of "mental illness" being *real* "illness" comes out in bold relief. Not only law grants the right to choose mental healthcare via myriad medical options, it claims to create a range[65] of medical options, all under the umbrella of biomedical psychiatry!

Take for instance Section 21 of the Act. Right to equality and non-discrimination suggests since mental illness is just another "illness" psychiatric "patients" should be treated like any other patients and all facilities given to any patient be extended to psychiatric "patients". Some of these services are (i) no discrimination,[66] (ii) emergency facilities and emergency services,[67] (iii) ambulance services[68] and (iv) medical insurance.[69]

For a patient the choice of treatment is their own decision, whether allopathy, *ayurveda*, macrobiotics or anything else. Whether or not the individual wants treatment is also a matter of their judgement, true for all patients. If psychiatric "patients" are at par with other patients they deserve the same freedom of choice, including whether or not they wish to be "treated". Whatever they decide thereafter has to be accepted as their preferred option with no insistence on a particular form of treatment. Merely creating parity with no options to choose between, without acknowledging that the individual deciding for herself is legally at par with others: (a) having legal soundness of mind and (b) capability to take action for herself, is but an empty shell. This creates other means to circumscribe people within the psychiatric system by any means, whether by giving access to ambulance or insurance. Thus the MHCA foists psychiatric knowledge as *the truth*, creating in response to the truth means to act upon it. The underlying assumption, which started from the first mental health legislation in 1858

---

64 MHCA, Section 18: Every person shall have a *right to access mental healthcare* and treatment from mental health services run or funded by the appropriate Government (emphasis supplied).
65 MHCA, Section 18, Subsection (3).
66 MHCA, Section 21, Subsection (1a).
67 ibid, Subsection (1b).
68 ibid, Subsection (1c).
69 ibid, Subsection (4).

continues to determine the fate of psychiatric "patients" albeit in the garb of "progress".

This arrangement of giving parity to psychiatric "patients" with others is particularly disturbing as it encourages the belief that people have real psychiatric emergencies for which they need ambulances to be taken to hospitals. The truth[70] is that whenever an ambulance is called for a psychiatric "patient" it is an act of coercion against the person, a colluded rejection of their *will and preferences* at work. The collusion is between family and psychiatrists, for which the State brings its force to back their decision, via legalized ambulance services and personnel capable of exerting force. If not coercion what would hold back a psychiatric patient from walking up to the ambulance, for they do not have a walking problem at all! An ambulance for a mental health issue is nothing but overt coercion, both illegal and violating people's rights and legal capacity. By expanding the means to control, medicate, take them against their will by ambulances and emergency services, psychiatric "patients" stand little chance for recovery. In fact it amounts to a further enmeshment with the system. Overall such coercive "treatments" can only be more traumatic and drive people into greater distress than relieving any. With this clause, psychiatric professionals stand to recover whatever ground they ceded to the CRPD, not "patients".

Creating awareness about "mental illness"

MHCA, Section 30 is dedicated to making recommendations for "creating awareness about mental health and illness and reducing stigma associated with mental illness". This may be read as government expenditures in perpetuating psychiatric rhetoric! Let us examine extant studies in this field. "Anti-stigma efforts in recent years have often been predicated on the assumption that neuroscience offers the most effective tool to reduce prejudice and discrimination" (Pescosolido et al., 2010:1312). From a mixed methods study of the impact of one such campaign in rural Andhra Pradesh, India, Maulik et al. (2017) report:

> results suggest that the knowledge of the study participants about mental health did not differ significantly following the intervention, but both their attitudes and behaviours did change for the better in most situations. This is one of the few studies globally, which measured changes in behaviour using a set of questions

---

70 I have witnessed this personally, though only as a witness in another's case not myself personally and I have heard testimonies of many individuals, none of who are part of this research.

around hypothetical scenarios, although not in real-life situations. *Stigma towards accessing mental healthcare* was also reduced following the intervention.

(emphasis supplied)

This indicates that even though the knowledge of people did not change in any significant manner, at least their *readiness to accept psychiatric treatment did*. This is a contradiction to the goals of awareness about mental "illness" the CRPD proposes. One would ordinarily think that stigma reduction campaigns would be geared towards inclusion of the "mentally ill" in their communities. Their goals may be rehabilitation, or ending prejudice against those stigmatized. The truth, however, is nowhere close. These stigma reduction campaigns are *not* for inclusion of "patients", but for *acceptance of psychiatric knowledge as truth* for responding to human suffering, and spreading the notion that medical intervention provides the way out of deep distress for scores of people.

Constituting the central mental health authority

The MHCA created scope for establishing massive bureaucratic machinery for governing mental health of the Indian people and to ensure they can access mental health services. Two sets of organizations having large capacities to monitor service delivery, execution and accountability have been created at the national and state levels. These organizations are the Central[71] and State Mental Health Authority[72] in each state respectively. This meticulous attempt, wherein each aspect of these organizations are designed, funds allocated, personnel defined increase pathways through which psychiatric knowledge reaches the farthest, and deepest in society, becomes reified and normalized.

Several new groups, who previously had no representation in mental health related decisions, have been inducted in the running and management of mental health affairs in India. These groups include caregivers,[73] patients,[74] and a whole array of psy-professionals. By examining the categories of these recruitments, it is evident there are *few or none* capable of contributing to recovery as each of these groups are likely to accept and amplify psychiatric knowledge. It may be remembered from the earlier reference (Chap 4) that it is primarily caregivers who accompany their children to psychiatric clinics. When more such individuals intervene at executive levels

71 MHCA, Sections 33–44.
72 MHCA, Sections 45–56.
73 MHCA, Section 34 (1) clause (n).
74 MHCA, Section 34, Subsection (1), clause (m): two persons representing persons who have or have had mental illness, to be nominated by the Central Government as members.

or as pressure groups, they further reinforce psychiatric practices by demanding more services, and infrastructure. By propagating and advocating psychiatric ontology further and facilitating its wider spread, all hurdles to colonize larger numbers of people are removed in this organized manner. Full state machinery is activated to enable psychiatric "patienthood"!

Not to be missed people with lived experiences have been inducted into the Central and State mental health authorities as well. It raises suspicion behind this intent as their numbers are so small and manner of inclusion so opaque, in all likelihood they too would end up shoring psychiatric rhetoric. One is left wondering who such people could be and would they even be aware of their own colonization? Would they not be mere cogs in a pharma-driven machinery propagating a learnt, deficit-driven view of their life struggles recast as "illness" categories? I have already questioned the viability of "lived experience" for its knowledge claims (see Chapter 2) and who gets to represent such experience. Voronka (2016) warns about those who get recruited to occupy such positions for it would be people who already believe in psychiatric knowledge. Their presence in the CMHA would be only tokenistic.

More problematically while the recruitment of every other person is narrowly defined in terms of their degrees and official positions, people with lived experiences can be *anyone*: no requirement of education, prior work in mental health activism/scholarship or anything. The concern is since anyone may get recruited, regardless of ability to contribute meaningfully towards the interest of "patients", the effort is to prove to international organizations (CRPD, W.H.O. etc.) that people with "lived experience" have fair representations in India. If they have critical views they would be so small in numbers, vastly outnumbered by psychiatry's advocates that refuting the psy-leviathan would be beyond their capacity, more so if not backed by organizations but appearing as one-off individuals. To have the capacity to counter psychiatric propaganda one has to be well entrenched in critical perspectives, activism and scholarship at the same time, and have tremendous capacity to work towards creating the counter discourse, another humongous task impossible in the absence of resources.

It is due to activism of ex-patients, activists and survivors involved with formulation of the CRPD this heroic and prodigious battle was waged and people with lived experiences gained a representation on professional forums. Before the CRPD such self-representations of ex-/patients were neither legal nor considered epistemically viable. If "patient" representation on professional forums is largely by those who agree and further diffuse psychiatric knowledge it nullifies the gains for any contrarian views. Psychiatry would once again end up creating and sitting in its own echo chamber, with an array of courtiers. *This* is a reason that those who question psychiatric knowledge should be present in such governmental bodies – to facilitate democratic dialogue. However considering the size of the Central Mental Health Authority, in all likelihood, even if they are there such people would still suffer marginalization due to numerical insufficiency.

The Convention insists time and again that legal capacity of patients is non-negotiable. Yet in each provision of the MHCA there are few subsections or clauses where the "patient's" capacity can be challenged, negotiated, threatened, taken back or questioned. For legal capacity to be actualized a less bureaucratic structure is conducive, wherein individual cases do not go through a convoluted governmental process for redressal of wrongs. Giant enforcement structures belie concern for the individual. Their main challenge is how the law should be activated, the law that *does not support recovery*. This institution is created to accelerate dispersal of psychiatric "truth", not recovery outcomes, for that would necessitate an infrastructural approach with a radically different emphasis.

In the present constitution of the CMHA the manner of serving the interests of "patients" (assuming it is to recover) is questionable. This organization will consolidate the arm of psychiatry – to increase the reach of psychiatric medication further and wider; making more people debilitated and disabled over time!

Mental health policy, CRPD and the MHCA

Post-independence until 2014, India did not have a mental health policy even while it had mental health programs: the National Mental Health program since 1982 and District Mental Health Program since 1996 (Sarin and Jain, 2017). This indicates a lack of a long-term vision with respect to meeting the goals of mental health needs of the country note Sarin and Jain (ibid), and therefore the announcement of a policy may be considered a step in creating a unified vision for the whole country.

Notwithstanding other claims, about how it conceptualizes mental health, its executive summary reads as following:

> It is significant that the 65th World Health Assembly held in 2013 approved and adopted resolution WHA.65.4 on *global burden of mental disorders* (emphasis supplied) and the need for a comprehensive, co-ordinated response from the health and social sectors at the community level. This National Mental Health Policy is in consonance with the intent of this WHA Resolution.
>
> (MoHFW, 2014:2)

The Policy document (henceforth Policy) which was released in 2014 is called *New Pathways, New Hope* (ibid.) and appears to be a representative document involving all stakeholders. Its approach to mental health

175

seems proactive[75] and vision futuristic, on a first reading. It clearly spells the goal of Policy as being "to promote mental health, prevent mental illness, enable recovery from mental illness ... within a rights-based framework" (ibid:3).

The openness to approach adopted by the Policy was evident right from the beginning as the language in its Preamble also exhibits: "this policy is intended to be dynamic; all-encompassing and growing with regular review and feedback from people" (ibid:ii). It was not a fixed policy document which would remain unchanged for all times ahead, and from the beginning itself had an in-built scope for adaptability. Sarin and Jain (2017:705) confirm,

> [t]he way that society views mental health and illness, and the primacy it gives to privileging individual rights (as distinct from the rights of families or care givers, or, perhaps, those of communities) needs to be considered and articulated in both legislation and policy.

This was evident at least in the policy which signifies both (a) recovery and its facilitation and (b) the rights of people directly affected to be centralized in the approach towards mental health in society.

Conception of "rights"

In the segments on CRPD and MHCA, the nature of rights granted to individuals by each of these instruments is detailed. While the former recognizes legal capacity, making allowances for a person's expressed *will and preference*, the latter simply wants to give people a "right" to mental health, whose definition is determined by normative biomedical categories. So how can these two rights based perspectives, whose goals, methods and intentions are contradictory, align without one being subsumed under the other? In the Policy such clear cut description of rights is not evident.[76] Instead the Policy suggests *discussions* on the same!

---

75 Especially a statement like – "Policy ... acknowledges the significance and importance of relevant and useful local knowledge and practices ... along with ground realities and variations of the Indian context" (MoHFW, 2014:1).

76 "Violation of their rights is a common reality for persons with mental health problems. The design and implementation of policies, programmes and services for persons with mental health problems should therefore, be based on a rights-based perspective. Respecting the rights of persons with mental health problems will reduce stigmatizing and discriminatory behaviours. This Policy envisages that there be more discussions in public space on Rights of persons with mental health problems and in design of a system that upholds their rights." (MoHFW, 2014:7).

The spirit of democracy visible in widespread participation of stakeholders in policymaking was not visible when policy became law.[77] The law was, yet again, anchored in the Indian Lunacy Act of 1912, carrying shadows of the past and formulated primarily by psychiatrists.[78] Whenever psychiatric knowledge is privileged over another epistemic framework certain ideas have to be foregrounded. First, psychiatry has historically maintained that "mental illness" is real "illness"; a claim (largely) unquestioningly accepted by a range of stakeholders.[79] Based on this it has time and again proposed medical "treatments", reinforcing prejudicial and stereotypical representation of "patients" with attributes such as "incompetence, dangerousness to self and others" (Dhanda, 2018:394).

Since the Policy document is explicit it is in consonance with WHA 65.4 it necessitated an inquiry. "In May 2012 the World Health Assembly adopted resolution WHA 65.4", notes Ivbijaro (2012), "and charged the World Health Organization (WHO) with the development of an action plan to respond to this". In response, the WHO came up with the zero draft of the Global Mental Health Action Plan 2013–2020.

> The zero draft of the Global Mental Health Action Plan 2013–2020 proposes a global vision and some core principles including universal access and equity in mental health; the promotion of human rights; the application of evidence-based practice; the adoption of a life course approach; the adoption of a multi-sectoral approach and the empowerment of people with mental disorders.
>
> (ibid)

I studied the zero draft of the Global Mental Health Action Plan 2013–2020 to examine what recommendations were made to individual nations and how rights of "patients" were defined.[80] The document has a time frame which "covers the period from 2013 to 2020. Within this period, intermediate targets are also specified"[81] (W.H.O., 2012:6). The first

---

77 For instance Sarin and Jain (2017:720) note that the "policy writing process has been, at least in some ways, a departure from earlier ... the first attempt at incorporating different stakeholder perspectives in policy-making, and, also, in a sense, has encouraged wider consultative participation".

78 A detailed exposition of this process is offered by Dhanda (2018).

79 Until the CRPD the "patients" could not directly contribute to this process. The CRPD has enabled that participation and contribution. In all mental health legislations prior to the CRPD "patients" had no representation. It is only after 2008 that their voices have become audible, though still quite marginal.

80 I have noted some of the recommendations in footnote 85.

81 The Global Mental Health Action Plan will have the following objectives: (1) To strengthen effective leadership and governance for mental health (2) To provide comprehensive, integrated and responsive mental health and social care services in community-based settings

objective of this document was strengthening governance in mental health-care, which has been accomplished in India by the MHCA. The next objective[82] is more explicit about "patients", yet little has been included in Indian Policy. It appears the Policy document in India adopted certain ideas for the Indian milieu and left the rest out.

There is precious little in the Indian law or policy which can support people's recovery. Since these instruments are predicated on psychiatric ontology and epistemology, the right to access biomedical treatments is entrenched in the system, *not right to recover or heal*. Still it does not foreclose the option of people recovering: for those who have enabling support from their environments, are personally tenacious, continue rehabilitation, quit psychiatric medication can circumvent the barriers to recovery.

My goal in this chapter was to examine the three instruments – the Convention, MHCA and Policy to see which of these would enable or catalyse recoveries, and whether any impedes. It seems evident while the Convention has created scope to support people's recoveries in diverse ways, the MHCA and Policy have not followed suit, choosing to align with biomedical goals. It may be apparent that law has become the meta-barrier to recovery: it both promotes psychiatrization of people's distress via institutional mechanisms, and harbours micro-barriers within its folds where the day-to-day micro-politics of mental health plays out between patients, caregivers and psychiatrists.

---

(3) To implement strategies for mental health promotion and protection, including actions to prevent mental disorders and suicides (4) To strengthen information systems, evidence and research for mental health (WHO, 2012:6).

82 Community-based service delivery needs to go beyond the provision of medical treatment to encompass a recovery-based approach that puts the emphasis on supporting individuals with mental health problems to achieve their own aspirations and goals to lead fulfilling lives in the community. Since many persons with mental disorders experience high unemployment levels, lower educational levels, homelessness, poverty, isolation and a lack of integration within communities, services will need to support individuals, at different stages of the life course and as appropriate, to access employment, housing, educational opportunities, and to engage in community activities and programmes.

More active involvement and support of service users in the reorganization and actual delivery of services is required, so that care and treatment become more responsive to the needs of persons with mental disorders and their carers. Greater collaboration with "informal" mental health care providers, as well as religious leaders, school teachers, police officers and local NGOs, is also needed. These groups can receive information about different types of mental health problems, their effects on individuals, and how to effectively assist and support people with mental disorders (ibid:.7).

7

DECOLONIZING
RECOGNITION

A person is a political being ... in the larger sense of political,
equal to other individuals, with rights, obligations, and the
ability to redress injury by others and by the state. Sickness
can interfere here, producing the fear of political powerless-
ness and lack of representation ... All relationships between
people ... are relationships of power; of subordinance, domi-
nance, or equipotence. The powerlessness of the sick person's
body and the ability of others to control the person by con-
trolling the body are part of the political dimension of illness.
(Cassell, 1991:41)

To reach the present stage of this winding road has taken three decades.
Where I stand the wasteland has been painstakingly explored, dwelled
in, meditated, reflected upon, crossed, revisited, and its milestones recognized. One cannot but begin with the disquieting recognition of those lost
in the labyrinth, helplessly waiting to be devoured by the Minotaur.[1] The
Minotaur is the psy-pharma complex which having created a tangled quag-
mire of ideas, deafening rhetoric and patriarchal discourse makes recovery
and exit near impossible for each who goes in. Those seeking biomedical
solutions for their distress, majority among them youth, enter newer ending "treatment" regimens and the Daedalian[2] maze of the Pharmageddon
(Healy, 2012). To exit the puzzle, one may have to be a slayer – who can
vanquish old ideas, and dare to look for a way out, even in haze.

---

1 In Greek mythology, the Minotaur was a monster with the body of a man and the head and tail
   of a bull. The Minotaur was the offspring of the Cretan Queen Pasiphae and a majestic bull.
   Due to the Minotaur's monstrous form, King Minos ordered the craftsman, Daedalus, and his
   son, Icarus, to build a huge maze known as the Labyrinth to house the beast. The Minotaur
   remained in the Labyrinth receiving annual offerings of youths and maidens to eat. He was
   eventually killed by the Athenian hero Theseus. For further details: https://www.worldhistory.
   org/Minotaur/.
2 Refer to footnote 1.

DOI: 10.4324/9781003248804-9   179

Theseus, the hero-slayer of the Minotaur, entered Crete from without, as the symbol and arm of the rising civilization of the Greeks. That was the new and living thing. But it is possible also for the principle of regeneration to be sought and found within the very walls of the tyrant's empire itself.

Campbell (2008:12)

Theseus – the slayer of the Minotaur, in this case can assume any face among the varied stakeholders of this puzzle, though "patients" or peers may constitute a majority. But each one troubled by the psy-pharma incestuous relationship can well be the slayer of the monster; whether caregivers, activists, critical thinkers, academics, psychiatrists or other psy-professionals. It all depends upon who has cultivated the capacity for such critique, and suspicion of hegemonic claims. For us this is an opportunity to revisit the labyrinth we navigated thus far, to mark its signposts.

Where lay barriers to recovery

Barriers to recovery principally lie in three relational domains, amidst intrapersonal and intersocial spaces. As Cassell (1991) notes interactions between people are based on a power differential which determines whether power or its lack is entrenched further or overcome; barriers erected or surmounted. I distinguish the former to be lying in micro- and macro-domains of sociality. Critical discourse analysis (Chapter 4) explicates how a person's reality is sidestepped when she accepts the "truth" of the "patient" role. This reality soon leads to her self-reassessment as a "mentally ill" subject, and her identity now a stigmatized one, becomes both a source of mortification and an intrapsychic barrier to recovery.

Stigma as barrier: Stigma impedes recovery in two ways. The social stigma faced by individuals and their families is the first, and the self-stigma "patients" internalize the second stigma-related barrier. In their hence reconfigured future, this self-directed stigma, accompanied by a sense of helplessness and loss of self-worth, becomes the first level of barrier. The ability to deal with stigma is a related and necessary condition for recovery; else stigma can overwhelm the bearer of a devalued social identity, pushing them into greater withdrawal and alienation from the world around them.

Micro-politics of mental health: Parents, among other caregivers, often become agents of psychiatry in domestic spheres. Within this relational triad – of "patient", caregiver and psychiatrist, the micro-politics of mental health plays out. Its focus is on governing the "patient", ensuring drug compliance and adherence to psychiatric recommendations in letter and spirit. Their chief purpose is to *manage* the "patient" accomplished by minor spoken words or queries about medication. Thus the "patient's" autonomous decision making ability doesn't emerge and frequent monitoring disallows them from developing a matured response to challenges of living; their efforts thwarted by the watchful, panopticonic gaze of the caregiver and/or psychiatrist.

Agency by itself is not adequate to ensure recovery; it requires further support to exit psychiatric medication, including contiguous rehabilitation measures and affirmative family support. Recoveries occur as a combined outcome of these variables *beyond the psychiatric gaze*, for continuing psychiatric medication itself is an obstacle, or worse – a cause for disability (Appendix C).

Largely two of the three barriers are visibly relational; how a "patient" relates with herself and others relate with her. The first barrier (internalized) stigma creates helplessness, while the second barrier microenvironment confines the individual within the psychiatric spectrum of ab/normalcy. Yet barriers are not neatly confined to micro-environments alone. They emanate from a bigger dimension: the meta-dimension of law and policy.

Legal-policy barriers: While the role of law is to create frameworks for governing citizens and ensuring their rights, it also adjudicates on what such rights should be. It appears reasonable that the "patient's" right maybe *right to heal or recover.* So why does law simplistically recognize suffering as "illness", push the individual into interminable "treatments", not healing or recovery? Don't interminable "treatments" prolong suffering? How does it reflect on law? Is the law misguided, misinformed about the purported nature of psychiatric "illness" or simply indifferent? Does the role of law in mental health remain confined to creating structures of governance for managing "mentally ill" subjects? If so in what manner is the law different from colonial laws which created segregated institutions for isolating "such (dangerous) people" in the "interest" of individual and society? This prejudicial visualization of the individual betrays their right to liberty and equality as citizens, while reducing them to governable "others" whose will and preferences matter but little. If the laws of a sovereign nation grants identical rights to citizens as former colonial masters what is the relevance of constitutional freedoms? Do they even exist for the "mentally ill"?

The **UN-CRPD** created an array of rights for persons with disabilities, which once ratified by State Parties became a legal commitment in respective jurisdictions. While these rights did not specifically mention goals of recovery the Convention still created several mechanisms which recognize the capacity of an individual to make judgements for herself and choose between treatment options or not choose any. Yet the MHCA, promulgated years after the CRPD, quietly shoved those rights away.

A grave injustice occurred in a quiet manner for gains made by prolonged efforts of disability activists globally: freedoms and liberty gained were subverted by how the MHCA legislated in favour of psy-professionals. It surreptitiously turned all rights of PwD/"patients" over to professionals by inserting small subsections and clauses within the Act that ensured egalitarian ideas: *legal capacity* and *will & preference* dispensable, making the Act practically useless for the "patient".

The overturning dismantles gains from the CRPD and ends up creating a convoluted maze of psychiatric "treatments" from which few will find a way out. Recovery would be a chance due to individual circumstance or disposition, similar to some peer narratives in this book. The vast majority who embark upon the "patient" role are unlikely to recover and will possibly progressively become enfeebled. The MHCA by reifying psychiatric ontology has created a massive governance structure, causing grievous harm, more injurious than any other barrier.

My goal of recognizing barriers to recovery lies fulfilled to the extent feasible. The next goal for this book is....

Instituting recovery

The idea of recovery belongs to the future for a majority. Instituting evidence of recovery became a key task when I embarked on this road, in 2011, documenting my recovery. When it failed its desired outcomes, and an opportunity to re-analyse recovery appeared it brought me to peer-research. Many overcome psychiatric constructions and create self-defined goals and futures (see Chapter 5). From that analysis, I propose recovery as a two-stage process, confirmed in mine and other narratives, equally having resonance among most "ex-patient" recovery narratives. These stages are:

i   **Become free from psychiatric medication** – the psychiatric past is left behind and the individual becomes functional in daily living, by becoming an active agent of self-transformation. Someone may initially, even periodically, rely on psychiatric medication, but in time find and/or create other means to go off medication.

ii **Developing agency and insight** to understand challenges of life and distress, gaining a sensibility to look beyond psychiatric diagnostic categories and learning to see personal problems in their larger social and structural origins. Instead of looking within oneself and bemoan a chemical imbalance start looking outside in the familial and sociological contexts.

Stages of recovery build one upon another and rest on people's agential capacity, which develops over a span of persistent effort. In a *drug-free recovery paradigm* people play an agential role themselves, with little/no guidance from psychiatrists. If any, it comes from other sources of healing they choose themselves. Those fully recovered recognize recovery as a stage of moving beyond psychiatric dependence, leaving "patienthood" behind and "gaining autobiographical power" (Myers & Ziv, 2016). While psychiatry-led recovery may involve both clinical and personal variants, the latter being an adjunct to the former (Harper and Speed, 2012:13) an emancipatory view envisions recovery as a liberatory exercise: recovery from psychiatry, and subjecthood!

I propose personal recoveries as catalysed by micro-environments when they do not act at the behest of psy-discourses and support the surfacing of someone's agency. Alternately, caregivers and psy-professionals jeopardize people's chances of accomplishing full scale recoveries (Chapter 4). All recoveries exhibit following attributes:

a   **Recovery outcome of rehabilitation choices** – Nobody who recovers sets recovery as a goal in the beginning; all try different ways to rehabilitate and deal with their distress. They take responsibility by disallowing a temporary setback to permanently derail their life and futures.

b   **Discontinuing psychiatric medication** – Each individual discontinues psychiatric "treatment" and accomplishes *drug free personal recovery*, not psychiatry-led *clinical recovery*.

c   **Individual agency** – Individuals themselves are agential and unfettered in making choices, personally becoming agents of change. Certain individuals like Rupali and Akshay, also vehemently oppose psychiatric medication.

d   **Supportive families** – Though all families respond in the same manner when faced with an "emergency" eventual recovery outcome(s) also emerge due to their catalysing role. While a majority seeks psychiatric support accompanied by someone from the family,[3] the latter being the first support system for most, un/knowingly and/or unwillingly they can become agents of subjectivation. Rupali's and Akshay's narratives exhibit possibilities when "patients" oppose medication and there is no coercion for compliance from the family. Such individuals can recover fully in a relatively shorter time.

Since the key goals of this book have been addressed, the question becomes what takes time to understand? Why do people, including me when similarly placed, not understand the issue or for what reason were we ignorant so long? Isn't it our task to probe.

Why recognition matters

Recognition spreads across diverse terrains in this book. From psychiatric *misrecognition* of distress as "illness", the path towards undoing it is

---

3 I have clarified in Chapter 4 that even if initially people do not go to a psychiatrist but seek other support, at some point all systems become conduits that bring people into the psychiatric fold.

traced, with possibilities for reclamation of life beyond psychiatric control. Layers of recognition blur into one another: from recognition of the need for "care" construed as "treatment" to a biomedical causality of unrecognizable behaviours. There is a possibility of a recognition in the "patient" about prognosis or a need to look beyond psychiatry, or an eventual discernment, wherever such agency is feasible that the initial recognition was a *misrecognition*, or at least insalubrious! One is tempted to ask about psy-professions, "[a]re their ways of parsing health phenomenon useful (Richardson, 2020:140)?" There is also a sobering recognition that mental health legislation, notwithstanding rhetoric and claims of progressiveness are in fact quite the opposite: reifying diagnosis and entrenching status quo while rights of "patients" safeguarded by CRPD stand surreptitiously undermined.

Is not politics of recognition the heart of the matter – who recognizes whom, towards what end? Does not the recognition by the sufferer, of the professional, mislead them? Yet, what else can they do in the absence of other healing options? Does the professional's recognition relieve suffering? Or does it push people towards further suffering? So what is law doing and what are psy-professions aiming at? Do they have no idea their solutions are inefficacious? They appear to simply colonize the mind as though giving a better, scientific or objective explanatory framework, instead causing grievous harm?

It is clear about the professional's recognitions that "patienthood" helps maintain their professional claims, and ensure social status, dominance and viability. "Patients" have to question whether it serves any purpose to be recognized thus. What needs to be recognized?

Representation: care or coloniality?

Does any form of care have to reduce the cared-for to an object? If a professional group is so adept, why is there a desire to control anyone? Wherefrom comes the need to create structures of governance, as though those governed need such violence in their "own best interest"? Why not simply create options, let people choose for themselves? Is this really caring or another form of coloniality?

Looking back a troublesome issue is the dilemma of representations (Chap 1): why do some representations carry more salience, and how can those with emancipatory agendas counter such dominance? There is lack of clarity about diagnosis yet people get routinely diagnosed and "treated". In a social ecology where "our epistemic lives are interdependent" (Pohlhaus, 2014:100), certain epistemic claims are privileged and others lack testimonial credibility. In denying people an epistemic agency testimonial injustice unfairly excludes particular epistemic agents from participating fully in this most basic of social epistemic practices based on an unwarranted, but widely held, identity prejudice, we can see that it constitutes an epistemic wrong (ibid: 101).

This writing has arisen from the bottom of the heap, by a voice representing the violence unleashed on a segment of humanity by the social power of coloniality. I do not seek permission to speak as the subaltern – I simply do. My self-assurance obscures my vulnerability: the need is not just to be heard but understood. To communicate we all need an audience willing and capable of hearing us. The extent to which entire populations of people can be denied this kind of linguistic reciprocation as a matter of course institutes epistemic violence (Dotson, 2011:238).

This book has tried challenging the pervasive (epistemic) harm to "patients" by recognizing their narratives as truth bearing and worthy of testimonial inclusion. In the process, it has laid bare the world of the "mentally ill" to help ascertain whether they who went seeking succour got relief, and raises the question whether it amounts to justice. "The most significant outcome of this revision or shift in perspective is that the agency of change is located in the insurgent or the 'subaltern'" (Spivak, 2010:330). The pinnacle of agency is visible in a few narratives (Chapter 5) where people recover beyond the psychiatric gaze, taking control of their lives, diagnoses, prognosis while their social contexts does not sabotage this emergence. The contrast is visible in a majority of others where "patienthood" is stable and people remain wedded to diagnostic identities.

This is the story of scores who do or will keep referring others to continue seeking this form of "relief", largely acting from, what may be construed, epistemic ignorance. But possibly ignorance may not entirely be the case – it may well be helplessness in the absence of alternatives. People only know of psychiatry from propaganda or the belief it offers "mind medicine". Whether or not "treatments" produce the relief they seek, the nature of prognosis and how one eventually recovers are areas of clear-cut ignorance. Issues of health and treatments remain shrouded in haze and belief in doctors supersedes all subjective outcomes, including comorbidities.

It is visible that recovery is feasible and many who don't recover may be really close. But not having a person, idea, institution or facilitation which can guide, help or assist them, nor having the agential capacity to counter hegemonic claims and fear which psy-rhetoric drives into people leave them with limited options except conceding to their "patienthood". Their inability is not necessarily a reflection on them but the prevalent culture, which stymies their efforts, nipping agency in the bud, augmented by psychiatry's "violently seized privilege behind a speciously rigorous scientism" (Richardson, 2020:132).

Analysis in preceding chapters shows interlocking variables of gender, marriage, patriarchy and school or university education as sources of deep distress. This is not a comprehensive picture for it does not account for age, poverty, language, religion, caste, homelessness, regionalism and scores of other variables which have similarly deleterious outcomes, not to forget the farm sector distress and suicides (see Aggarwal, 2008). "Culture ... is a legitimate, even necessary, terrain of struggle, a site of injustice in its own right and deeply imbricated with economic inequality" (Fraser, 2000:109). But the foundational issue is not even culture specific – it is more generic, ontological and ethical. It lies in the ethics of care and the "medicalization of ordinary life" (Frances, 2013).

Sholl (2017:266) refers to the "medicalization thesis" which has developed since the 1960s and 1970s due to the work done by sociologists, physicians and theorists such as Ivan Illich, Irving Zola, Thomas Szasz, Michel Foucault and later Peter Conrad and Joseph Schneider. This book aimed to capture how various conditions, behaviours or experiences which were previously under legal, political or religious surveillance, and as such were not "inherently medical", are becoming increasingly defined as medical entities to be labelled and treated. While Downing (in Sholl, ibid.) confirms that "[m]edicine used to claim authority over the cracks and interruptions in life; now it claims authority over all of life", Conrad (in ibid.) expands this proposition to suggest "the populace has internalized medical and therapeutic perspectives as a taken-for granted subjectivity". The medicalization thesis is a critique of the increasing footprint of medicine usage in daily life and

> to denounce various trends in twentieth-century (Western) medicine, such as the usage of medical categories and treatments to control deviant behavior, the widening of diagnostic categories ("disease mongering"), the commodification of health, the problem of iatrogenesis, the tendency to obscure the social or political context of illness, the privatization of medical practice, and the role of pharmaceutical companies in shaping diagnoses and treatments.
>
> (ibid:266–267)

Each of these aspects of medicalization is evident in the narratives of this book, a grim indicator it could be happening in diverse medical fields. When life is so medicalized where does the sufferer seek relief? Who can we expect justice from – the market, the pharmaceutical corporation, the doctor or law? Where does this recognition lead us?

Where do we go from here?

All of us come from some historical limitation, which cannot be overcome until recognized. Yet each carries a heroic potential to play their role creating minuscule change capable of causing further eddies. My orientation for this book as "future forming" comes from this location. The future I envision is based on a collaborative, polyphonic dialogue underpinned by commitment to epistemic plurality. Much as I wish to advance a resistance, I realize even among seemingly adversarial ranks there may be interlocutors, doubters, radicals and rejecters of psy-pharma practices. There is little doubt we, who have sought healing, have been profoundly wronged. We cannot but bemoan "the uncanny resonances of violence enacted through medicine" (Bartlett, 2021). But to hold individuals – professionals or caregivers unilaterally responsible may not help, especially because they may not have known better, or at least not mostly. In three decades of treading this terra firma, I have come across vastly different perspectives among all constituencies which make overarching generalizations untenable.

By recognizing this, I am not ready to surrender our resistance, or think we can start accepting colonial representations and practices as our saviours. Politics enters into people's lives without their knowledge or consent. While power inherent in human relationships plays a governance role of "patients" most remain unaware of the invisible realm of its working. Nevertheless, everyone is acutely aware of their lack of power or inescapability from its control. The intention here is without giving up our efforts for epistemic justice, plurality and recognition we at least win over those who are already on the margins and willing to make the emancipatory turn towards the colonized, who look for the decolonial perspective equally like us. This leads us to the possibility of epistemic reformation and decolonizing epistemology.

What can be done?

Since the earliest recorded histories, writing or inscribing the law has been a political enterprise, and rulers have taken great pains to ensure that people will read the law and learn how to comply with its authoritative mandates (Jasanoff, 2011:1). "Political power", says Locke (1690/2012:4), amounts

> to be a right of making laws with penalties of death, and consequently all less penalties ... and of employing the force of the community, in the execution of such laws ... and all this only for the public good.

From this perspective of creating laws, no question arises that laws which have been created for the "mentally ill" are only for their "good", and mechanisms of governance thus created part of "their welfare". Do legislators making laws understand what is "best" or the machinery that watches over their implementation? A law created with such goals seems to be on "the mission to spread civic virtue with military power" (Gyan Prakash, 1995:4). How "helpful" can such a top down approach be for someone's healing or recovery?

If law only legitimizes medical "treatments", is it not complicit in per-petuating a wrong? What room does this leave for epistemic plurality if only medical treatments are mandated? Drawing on available evidence Davar and Lohokare (2012:274) point out "the positive aspects of healing and recovery through holistic methods in the shrines that offer social and safe spaces for experiencing life at moments of vulnerability and crisis". Is the law also willing to accommodate a perspective as subjective as this? Or would it act in someone's "best" interest, decide they deserve medical "treatment"? The moot question is *who decides what is "best"*? How does such law differ from the colonial master who considered it his moral re-sponsibility to civilize the "native" by framing their lives in modernist and "civilized" terms?

Does the "patient" need laws to govern her "treatment" or continuation within the mental health system? Or is law meant to ensure the "patient" gets to choose between recovery options? Or does the professional, who manages to convince the "patient" (Bossema et al., 2011) or caregivers (Pitschel-Walz et al., 2006) via psycho-education, about treatments and their efficacy, require the law more: to ensure compliance of "patients"? Assuming the "patient" needs the law, then who should define the terms of the law – the one whose economic interests are tied to it or the one in whose service the law is created? And if it is the former, could any among them be involved in the framing of such a law?

These questions need not be limited to law alone but can be asked of every stakeholder, in particular the professional – what do they want, at what cost and what means? Having gone the length of decoding barriers and demystifying treatments the question is *can the future remain more of the same* – where people who do not have basic health facilities are given mental health "treatments", when sanitation and food security are missing and maternal and infant mortality are rampant we give women treatments for their depressions, traumas and stresses trying to ensure the status quo of family and society, without concern for the person? And a similar injustice can be repeated for every demographic, and for how long? Is it not time to look for a new equilibrium?

Visualizing possibilities, framing futures

> Properly conceived, struggles for recognition can aid the redistri-bution of power and wealth and can promote interaction and co-operation across gulfs of difference.
>
> (Fraser, 2000:109)

Fraser's proposition opens a pathway of resistance for each who sees the inherent injustice and coloniality of psychiatric ontology "to make this epistemic violence legible" (Wispelwey, 2021:298). The future begins from a capacity for inverting the gaze and questioning who this ontology assists, or how; each individual and group having freedom to assess it for themselves. Only such a beginning would be germinal for a new future. It may necessitate many a rectification touching legal and policy reform, epistemic polyphony, decolonizing knowledge and health practices and lived experience's inclusion and scope for leadership (Bryne et al., 2018). While each of these have their unique challenges and ways of response my goal for now is only where we – former and current patients and Mad scholars could go, among other possibilities. For this, I lean into Mignolo's conceptual formulations to explain and describe colonial knowledge practices and anti-colonial epistemic resistance, built from Foucault's epistemic assessments of hegemony seeking versus subjugated knowledges (Alcoff, 2007:80).

Earlier (see Chapter 2) I posed the question if everything is a social construction can we reject the psychiatric alternative, in favour of a new construction? How easy will it be for those labelled "mad" to create an alternative social construction? Walter Mignolo and other Latin American philosophers have pointed out the hierarchical patterns of epistemic judgement under colonial systems (Alcoff, 2007:81). Leopoldo Zea (in ibid) says that

> the identity, the rationality, and the very humanity of the peoples … were put on trial and judged by the jury of its conquerors … (the former) were not considered to be in a position to present their own epistemic credentials, much less to judge European ones.

To make this clearer, it is not knowledge alone, derived from certain epistemic principles and practices that matters, but extra-epistemic concerns of race, and nationality which determine which knowledge can stake credibility. If Indian psychiatrists or psy-professionals from any erstwhile colony, or country of the Global South decided, they wanted to create an alternative system how readily will it be adopted? "Geo-politics of knowledge goes hand in hand with geo-politics of knowing. Who and when, why and where is knowledge generated (rather than produced, like cars or cell phones)?" (Mignolo, 2009:2).

Is it any coincidence those who gain visibility and voice in their home countries (of the Global South) position themselves in prominent locations in the Global North? It is from there that they leverage their "concern" for their countrymen, from amidst the erstwhile (plundering) colonizer by representing their modernist knowledge as a befitting response to injustices of life in the poverty-ridden Global South. They need to be seen in those galleries of power – as agents of "Modernity", offering solutions and explanatory frameworks that ride over our subjectivities as claims of *truth* and *objectivity*. When within psychiatry colonization dominates for ex-/"patients" to claim epistemic agency is nothing if not threatening. Morrison (2008:xi) also warns "[m]ental patients who resist treatment and insist on speaking for themselves against mental health practices are particularly feared and misunderstood".

Much of Mignolo's analytics of epistemology concerns its role in creating, developing and maintaining a hierarchy of knowledge and knowers particularly adapted for colonialism, in which the most relevant distinction concerned one's cultural identity (Alcoff, 2007:82). If my aim via this writing is to create an alternative, decolonial[4] way of looking at issues psychiatry deems "pathological" as being *issues of distress which the sufferer cannot communicate*, will it be recognized legitimate or would my position evoke prejudice, undermining my epistemic credibility?

Are contemporaneous generations of psy-professionals not playing the same colonial role by acquiring these tools (knowledge and methods of the human mind) of "Modernity" eschewing the need to ameliorate suffering from an ethical stance of care, justice and humaneness? Perhaps it would be best to leave this dilemma to the conscience of the individual professional to think for herself and have the moral courage to counter such claims to Modernity.

Whither resistance?

Perhaps my final goal for this writing is to consolidate the resistance of peers by offering certain ideas I could unravel. It neither summarizes our struggles, ends our resistance, nor can it foresee or predict what pathways lay ahead. It is to create a scope for further reflections and possible ways of thinking, at least through our immediate realities and throw light on the micro- and macro-variables that govern our bodies and minds. We need to comprehend more deeply the nature of emancipatory struggles and why an epistemological decentering is required. Mignolo (in ibid: 86) recommends, "we need a more extensive period of epistemological reflection. We need to develop a decolonial critical theory that will be more thoroughly delinked from the contemporary variants of the modern imperial designs of the recent past". We also need to think more local, less global – and unlike the Global Mental Health Movement make no generalized claims about any peoples claiming to understand their reality better than them. This is equally true for "patients" and peer groups, for there are no homogeneous groups anywhere waiting for solutions from other groups.

Colonized people anywhere have won political freedoms by organized resistance and developing ideas and methods to oppose the colonizer.

---

4 polanco and X (2021) propose the idea of Andean decoloniality: dedicated to making visible the complex colonial foundations of the modern world as a way to situate alternative ways of knowing, being, relating, sensing, and doing as being as legitimate as Western European cultural practices.

We have to look into history to understand those struggles against extractive forces of coloniality, similarly empower ourselves with tools commensurate with this resistance. We will be required to build solidarities and make efforts to raise consciousness among peers who continue getting into, or remaining entrapped by widespread psychiatric propaganda. It is premature to think psy-professions will voluntarily give up their epistemic claims, permit displacement that "challenges the norms or conventions of a system" (Banerjee, 2021). Yet, we needn't forget that "entrenched conventionality is the bane of all human endeavours and especially of science, which is synonymous with progress" (ibid).

No doubt epistemic reformation is the path ahead – but we are *not* the ones to bring reform to psy-knowledge(s); it has to be psy-professions' internal challenge(s) of decolonizing their epistemology and practices. We instead have to think of a wider struggle, beyond psychiatry, which embraces life in its social, economic and structural totality. We could think of social ecosystems where seeds of people's distress lurk and day-to-day injustices or oppressions take away the vitality of life in different ways, silencing the experiencer, obfuscating the experience into something unrecognizable, unthinkable yet governable. The activism of former patients and those opposing hegemonic knowledge claims must embrace wider struggles for justice, equality and democracy anywhere.

Appendix A
DEMOGRAPHIC PROFILES OF PEERS IN THIS BOOK

Status in the sequence: recovered (R), transitioning from "patienthood" (T) and "patients" (P). Names and locations are indicative of diversity yet occlude recognition (Table A.1).

Table A.1 Demographic profiles of peers as it appears in this book

Name (changed)	Status	Gender	Age at time of interview	Age at onset of psychosis	Diagnosis	Location	Caregiver who contributed
1. Rupali	R	F	41	25–26	Bipolar	NCR	Mother
2. Jitendra	R	M	60	18–19	Schizophrenia	West*	**
3. Akshay	R	M	30	25	Drug-induced psychosis	North*	Father
4. Sona	T	F	30		Bipolar	West*	Mother
5. Nithya	T	F	26	19	Bipolar	NCR	Mother and father
6. Hetal	T	F	24	20	Schizophrenia	NCR	Father
7. Vindhya	P	F	44	15–16	Schizophrenia	South*	**
8. Smita	P	F	45	16–17	Schizophrenia	West*	Father
9. Bhavna	P	F	47		Schizophrenia	NCR	Mother
10. Bharati	P	F	22	15	Schizophrenia	South*	Mother

*NCR stands for National Capital Region of Delhi. North, West and South indicate rough locations of cities on India's map.
**Caregivers of two individuals were not alive at the time of these interviews.

Appendix B

FLOWCHARTS

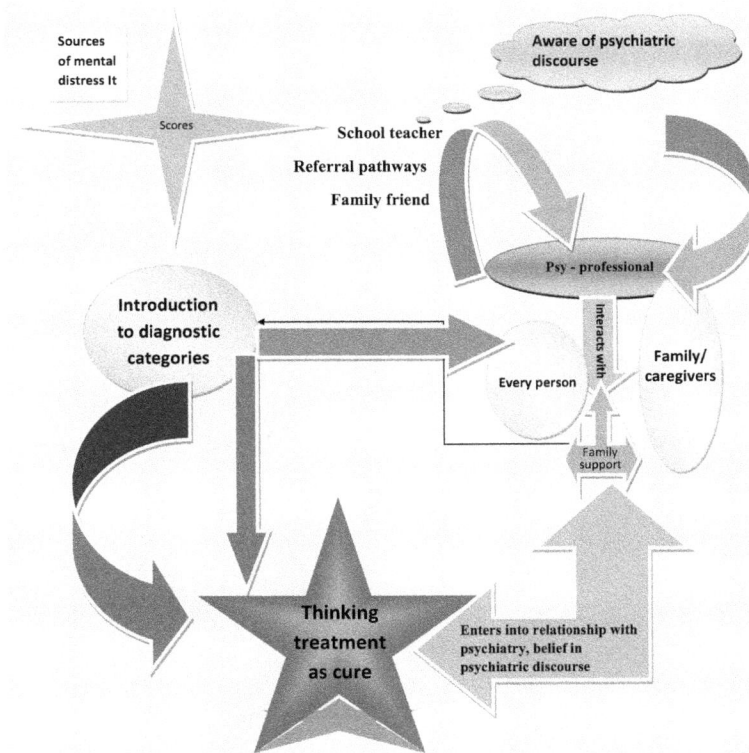

Flow chart A.1 Making of the psychiatric subject

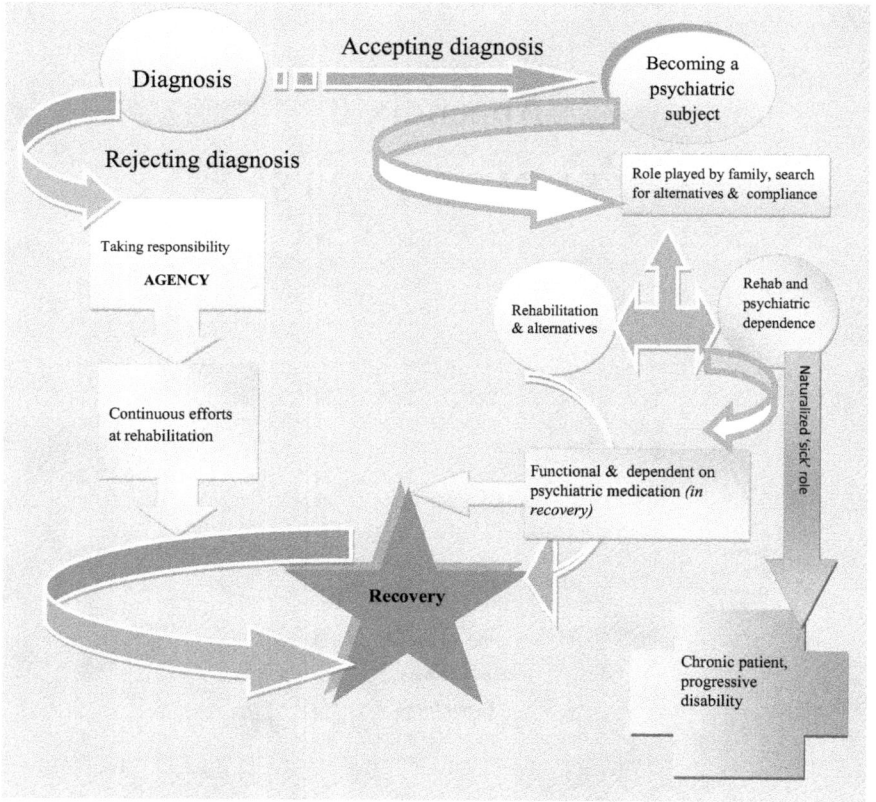

Flow chart A.2 Recovery in/from psychosis

Appendix C

FROM "TREATMENT" TOWARDS DISABILITY

Vindhya's unceasing neuroleptics[1]

A segment of Vindhya's narrative depicting the suffering of a chronic "patient" follows. She is resigned to her medical regimen, notwithstanding progressive debility. I extract from her narrative vignettes depicting several relationships – with her family, husband – when married, her psychiatrist and her ongoing "treatments". I offer no analysis but a factual illustration of matters as they stand. From there, I look for evidence in medical research of the outcomes due to her psychiatric treatment. My goal is to see how treatment impacts psychiatric "patients" in the long run and whether it assists dealing with life challenges any better than they could manage before they began or how close it takes them to recovery.

Vindhya started on psychiatric medication at age 15–16, as a school going youngster. At the time, I conducted this interview she was 44. Decades of psychiatric medication, marriage and divorce, family traumas including mother's death, brother's suicide, lack of regular involvement from her sister and her family who control her financial resources while not letting her stay with them have taken their toll. She feels vulnerable and uncertain about taking chances with anything new, notwithstanding setbacks being how she is.

ME: *"You won't recover... you believe that?"*
VINDHYA: *"Yes ma'am, I will not recover."*
ME: *"Because you have three diseases therefore you'll not recover, is that what (it is)?"*

---

1 Neuroleptics, also known as antipsychotic medications, are used to treat and manage symptoms of many psychiatric disorders. They fall into two classes: first-generation or "typical" antipsychotics and second-generation or "atypical" antipsychotics. Source: Ameer MA, Sangani A, Saadabadi A. Neuroleptic Medications. [Updated 2020 May 23]. In: StatPearls [Internet]. Treasure Island (FL): StatPearls Publishing; 2020 Jan. Available from: https://www.ncbi.nlm.nih.gov/books/NBK459150/. Accessed 18th June 2020.

VINDHYA: *"Yes ma'am, for Lupus doctor is telling... I myself don't know whether it will work out without the tablet, so you have to continue the tablets till your life ... end of the life".*
ME: "Yes?"
VINDHYA: *"So I am taking the tablets for Lupus"*

Vindhya was trained to be an engineer and she held a job before getting married. After marriage things became difficult *"Once he figured I was on medication his attitude towards me became very harsh, that made me quite depressed".*

In all my conversations,[2] whenever I encouraged her to step out and look for some work, she showed hesitancy in venturing out alone, until the side effects of lupus appeared in front of me. These side effects of psychiatric medication have debilitated her considerably, making her bowel movement unpredictable and a source of anxiety.

VINDHYA: *"But I cannot explain him (my psychiatrist) all this ... bowel problems and all I cannot explain."*
ME: *"Why? Why can't you explain?"*
VINDHYA: *"No ma'am, like even if I explain I ... once I ... I have told him once but he ... he forgot that ma'am."*
ME: *"He forgot?"*
VINDHYA: *"I told that... that I have a bowel problem".*

A background check of co-morbid conditions of systemic lupus erythematosus (SLE) with underlying psychiatric conditions reveals that "SLE is a chronic autoimmune disorder with occasional CNS manifestations. In a few situations, this disorder presents with psychiatric complaints but the psychotic features are infrequent" (Nayak et al., 2012).[3] In none of my dialogues with Vindhya have I ever heard her mention *any* "psychotic" conditions, or at least not the kind I have personally experienced! Yet she continues her medication and suffers increasing co-morbid conditions.

Since she is extremely cautious of venturing out, for fear of a sudden urge to empty her bowels, she remains increasingly confined at home. Her worst fear is a scenario wherein she cannot have access to a toilet when urgently needed. I further investigated the link between the

---

2 We have an ongoing association from November 2014, staying in touch on phone and WhatsApp. On her birthday, the new year and whenever there is a crisis we have long conversations. We try to look for solutions together, which often placates her momentarily; though she does not take initiative to launch into new things I egg her to try.

3 Nayak, R. B., Bhogale, G. S., Patil, N. M., & Chate, S. S. (2012). Psychosis in patients with systemic lupus erythematosus. *Indian Journal of Psychological Medicine*, 34(1), 90–93. https://doi.org/10.4103/0253-7176.96170.

prescribed medication (chlorpromazine) and her co-morbid conditions. First I looked for a link of her medication with lupus. The source[4] says that "[d]rug-induced lupus erythematosus is similar but not identical to systemic lupus erythematosus (SLE). It is an autoimmune disorder. This means your body attacks healthy tissue by mistake. It is caused by a re-action to a medicine". Chlorpromazine is listed as a possible drug that can cause SLE.

Her bowel sensitivity prompted me to examine the link between lupus and the gastrointestinal tract. Tian and Zhang[5] (2010) note

> Systemic lupus erythematosus (SLE) is an autoimmune inflamma-tory disease characterized by the presence of a plethora of auto antibodies and immune complex formation. Virtually every system and organ can be affected by SLE. Gastrointestinal symptoms are common in SLE patients, and more than half of them are caused by adverse reactions to medications and viral or bacterial infections. Though not as common as lupus nephritis, SLE-related gastrointes-tinal involvement is clinically important because most cases can be life-threatening if not treated promptly.

On tracing the development of her narrative, three stages stand out: (a) entry into the psychiatric system, (b) stabilizing with medication, no search for alternative, leading to first co-morbidity (lupus), (c) progressive dam-age to gastrointestinal tract due to lupus and fear of unexpected, untimely bowel movement, leading to social reclusiveness.

Since our association is now over seven years, I ask her about her medica-tion after a span of time and she confirms her "patienthood".

ME: *"Since you are a 'patient' how much medicine do you take... which makes you feel as a 'patient'?"*
VINDHYA: *"Medicines now...My psychiatric doctor has stopped all the medicines, he is giving medicine only for my sleep"*
ME: *"What medicine is that?"*
VINDHYA: *"I am taking Trinicalm Forte".*
R: *"Right, okay. So...".*
VINDHYA: *"I am taking one tablet of Trinicalm forte. That makes me sleep – for eight hours I can get sleep".*

---

4 https://medlineplus.gov/ency/article/000446.htm.
5 Tian, X. P., & Zhang, X. (2010). Gastrointestinal involvement in systemic lupus erythe-matosus: insight into pathogenesis, diagnosis and treatment. *World Journal of Gastroen-terology*, 16(24), 2971–2977.

I check again the uses and side effects[6] of the said drug. The website says:

> Trinicalm tablet falls under a category of drugs known as phenothiazine antipsychotics and is composed of Chlorpromazine, Trihexyphenidyl and Trifluoperazine. It is used as a psychiatric medicine. This medication treats mental and mood disorders such as bipolar disorder, ADHD and schizophrenia.

Its side effects are listed as dry mouth, nausea, vomiting and constipation. This information prompts towards further scrutiny, and I now search for long-term effects of anti-psychotic usage, without focusing on one drug. Correll, Rubio and Kane (2018)[7] suggest

> chronic antipsychotic use is associated with *metabolic disturbance* (emphasis supplied) and tardive dyskinesia. The latter is the clearest undesired clinical consequence of brain functioning as a potential result of chronic antipsychotic exposure, likely from dopaminergic hypersensitivity, without otherwise clear evidence of other irreversible neurobiological changes. Adjunctive psychosocial interventions seem critical for achieving recovery.

Strangely enough even though long-term effects of anti-psychotics are ambiguous, psychiatrists still do not hesitate to prescribe them,

> since there is strong evidence supporting efficacy of antipsychotics in reducing relapses over this time frame. Data on long-term outcomes are more equivocal and, although the effect of antipsychotics seems to decrease over time, this could be an artifact of long-term study designs.
>
> (ibid.)

"Mid-term" is anything between one and three years. But what about three decades?! And since there is no support from another therapeutic dimension, her life is caught between frames of psychiatric constructions.

Had Vindhya someone else around taking interest in her health and/or medical issues they may have challenged this unquestioned continuity of medication. But who can even say that now? There is no such person around; she lives alone in a big metropolis. This is not to say she has no social capital but the engaged attention a family's concern could engender is lacking. She continues getting into a deepening web of debility, worrying about her future, saying she is losing her memory every time we speak.

---

6 https://www.lybrate.com/medicine/trinicalm-forte-tablet.
7 Correll, C. U., Rubio, J. M., & Kane, J. M. (2018). What is the risk-benefit ratio of long-term antipsychotic treatment in people with schizophrenia? *World Psychiatry: Official Journal of the World Psychiatric Association (WPA)*, 17(2), 149–160. https://doi.org/10.1002/wps.20516.

Appendix D

THE HOMEOPATHIC MENTAL HEALTH ESTABLISHMENT

The position of homeopathy in integrated public health care is still an inadequately analysed area suggest Kaur, Chalia and Manchanda[1] (2019). Without exerting in that direction my goal for this appendix is to see what the philosophical basis of homeopathic treatment is, how it differs from allopathy or biomedicine (which is not modern or new) and what is the nature of work currently underway in homeopathy in the context of mental health. To respond to these queries, I first look at the principles of homeopathy as given by the founding father of homeopathy and then the current position of homeopathy in a mental health context. For the latter, I examine one institution marked as a national centre for research in homeopathy. I analyse their research and whether it is getting its due in the AYUSH department of the Government of India.

In his famous book *The Organon*, considered the cornerstone of homeopathic principles and practice, the founder of homeopathy Samuel Hahnemann (1842) notes,[2]

> [m]edicine as commonly practised (allopathy) knows no treatment except to draw from diseases the injurious materials which are assumed to be their cause ... Whenever it can, it employs, in order to keep in favor with its patient, remedies that immediately suppress and hide the morbid symptoms by opposition (contraria contrariis) for a short time (palliatives), but that leave the cause for these symptoms (the disease itself) strengthened and aggravated. It considers affections on the exterior of the body as purely local and existing there independently, and vainly supposes that it has cured them when it has driven them away by means of external remedies,

---

1 Kaur, H., Chalia, D.S., Manchanda, R.K. (2019). Homeopathy in public health in India. *Homeopathy*; 108(2): 76–87. DOI: 10.1055/s-0038-1673710.
2 Available at https://www.homeopathyschool.com/the-school/editorial/the-organon/authors-preface/, accessed on 11th June 2020.

so that the internal affection is thereby compelled to break out on a nobler and more important part.

With unusual prescience, as though foreseeing the birth of modern psychiatry, especially as it developed after the publishing of DSM-III (1980), Hahnemann further states,

> This non-healing art which for many centuries has been firmly established in full possession of the power to dispose of the life and death of patients according to its own good will and pleasure, ... (has in fact) in that period ... shortened the lives of ten times as many human beings as the most destructive wars, and rendered many millions of patients more diseased and wretched than they were originally.
>
> (ibid.)

Writing about the philosophical basis of how illness is treated in homeopathy, he notes further, as opposed to what he noted what the manner in which illness or disease was treated in the old system (allopathy, not included here),

> homoeopathy avoids everything in the slightest degree enfeebling, and as much as possible every excitation of pain, for pain also diminishes the strength, and hence it employs for the cure ONLY those medicines whose power for altering and deranging (dynamically) the health it knows accurately, and from these it selects one whose pathogenetic power (its medicinal disease) is capable of removing the natural disease in question by similarity (*simila similibus*), and this it administers to the patient in simple form, but in rare and minute doses so small that, without occasioning pain or weakening, they just suffice to remove the natural malady whence this result: that *without weakening, injuring or torturing him in the very least*, the natural disease is extinguished, and the patient, even whilst he is getting better, gains in strength and thus is cured – *an apparently easy* but actually troublesome and difficult business, and one requiring much thought, but which restores the patient without suffering in a short time to perfect health.

He concludes the preface to his book saying,

> Thus homoeopathy is a perfectly simple system of medicine, remaining always fixed in its principles as in its practice, which, like the doctrine whereon it is based, if rightly apprehended will be found to be complete (and therefore serviceable). What is clearly

pure in doctrine and practice should be self-evident, and all back-ward sliding to the pernicious routinism of the old school that is as much its antithesis as night is to day, should cease to vaunt itself with the honorable name of Homoeopathy.

I have given an extensive exposition of the underlying principles of home-opathy[3] to establish two things: (a) the basis on which it operates is funda-mentally different and somewhat opposed[4] to allopathy and (b) the focus of homeopathy when practiced correctly is to "cure" to produce healing without debilitating the "patient". It is not to "treat" interminably, the lat-ter operative in allopathy for centuries.

From this point, I would like to examine how the MHCA which created options of medical pluralism[5] came to look upon homeopathic institutions as "mental health establishments". National Homoeopathy Research Insti-tute[6] in Mental Health (NHRIMH), Kottayam, Kerala is the first Research institute in Homoeopathy under Central Council for Research in Homoe-opathy (CCRH), Ministry of AYUSH, Govt. of India. This was established in the year 1974 as Regional Research institute, later upgraded to Central Research institute for Homeopathy in 1982 and upgraded as NHRIMH in November 2016. *The main objective of the institute is to work for the de-velopment of Homoeopathic research and education* (emphasis supplied) ... The institute took further steps for the future development and envisaged its up gradation to the status of a national institute with a major objective to start PG degree programmes in Practice of Medicine and Psychiatry.

Homeopathy does not believe in isolating mental health issues from other health issues but in fact sees the individual as a whole that must be treated in her entirety.

It is first necessary to know that drugs can make man sick, and next to know what that state of sickness is. Every medicine that

---

3 In family homeopathy was practiced for two generations before me, my parental home replete with hundreds of books on the subject. My father practiced it once having a full dispensary. Though familiarity did not produce an urge to take it up professionally, it kindled recognition from allopathy early on. Yet this appreciation was not deep enough to trust my own healing with it when I was given a diagnosis and only after 18 years of psychiatric "treatment" when I found an elderly homeopath who told me I could be "fine" I reluctantly agreed to consider it. Such is the power of psychiatric propaganda that in spite of close proximity I never touched homeopathy nor my father pushed for it.

4 Samuel Hahnemann was a trained allopathic doctor, an M.D., before he took to inquir-ing into new ideas that eventually led to the development of homeopathy.

5 Cant (2020:1) defines it as "the coexistence of differing medical traditions and practices grounded in divergent epistemological positions and based on distinctive worldviews".

6 Taken from its website at: https://www.ccrhindia.nic.in/index1.aspx?lsid=433&lev=1&l id=371&langid=1&Regid=2, accessed on 11th June 2020.

a homoeopath uses should have been thoroughly proven upon the healthy so that its symptom image shall have been thoroughly brought out.

(Kent,[7] lecture 12)

This position is a contradiction to the clinical trials via which allopathic drugs are developed.

Mental health research at NHRIMH

The website of the NHRIMH informs,

till date Council has conducted 136 studies on various diseases, out of which 121 studies were concluded (106 were observational studies and 15 randomized clinical trials) and 15 studies were withdrawn. The salient achievements in clinical studies have been in HIV/AIDS, Acute Rhinitis in children, Gastroenteritis, Chronic Sinusitis, Influenza like illness, benign prostatic hyperplasia, acute haemorrhoids, cervical spondylosis pain management, urolithiasis etc.

Clearly mental health is not the sole occupation of this institution, even though it has been designated as a national centre for research in mental health. Their research shows a segment where data for all completed clinical studies can be downloaded. I examined this list to ascertain how many were conducted in mental health.

In a list of 156 studies, serial numbers 95–110 are assigned to psychiatric disorder (16 studies). Among these, four related to "schizophrenia", one discussed "acute mania", one study each was devoted to attention deficit hyperactivity disorder, autism, "psycho-physiological" disorders and depression, and seven studied behavioural disorders. This makes it a list of five in all relevant to the present work, among which I could access one.[8] This was a study of 171 patients given a "schizophrenia" diagnosis, who were visiting the NHRIMH. In the design section of this article, the authors note the following:

Each patient who presented with symptoms of schizophrenia was confirmed and *assessed by psychiatrist* at baseline and during follow-ups. *As guided by the psychiatrist* engaged in the study,

7 Accessed from http://www.homeoint.org/books3/kentlect/lect12.htm, accessed on 11th June 2020.
8 Oberai, P., Gopinadhan S., Sharma, A., Nayak C., Gautam, K. (2016). Homeopathic management of schizophrenia: A prospective, non-comparative, open-label observational study. *Indian J Res Homeopathy*; 10: 108–118. DOI: 10.4103/0974-7168.183877.

patients who showed "inadequate response to at least two 3rd generation antipsychotic drugs at the maximally tolerated dose within the recommended therapeutic range lasting 3 weeks" were considered as *treatment resistant cases.* Patients who had not taken antipsychotic treatment for the disease prior to enrolment were considered as "untreated cases." ... *The patients who were on antipsychotic drugs were allowed to continue the same along with homoeopathic medicines,* and the *dose of the same was monitored by the psychiatrist*; however, others were *prescribed homoeopathic medicines only as guided by the psychiatrist.*

(Oberai et al., 2016:109) (emphasis supplied)

The whole approach to homeopathy in this case appears to be guided by a psychiatrist, as though without such guidance homeopathy is not viable enough to manage "schizophrenia". One is left wondering how one expects a psychiatrist, trained in another epistemological and ontological view, to guide another in a wholly different epistemic location. If one were to refer back at the philosophical basis of homeopathy, the purpose of the whole exercise of allopathy guiding homeopathy for treatment appears to be self-defeating, farcical and questionable.

Homoeopathic treatment is the most curative, non-toxic, gentle and modern treatment. In view of the fact that it works with the person's own vital force towards equilibrium and healing, it will influence the brain chemistry and assist the patient in resuming psychological strength and symmetry.

(Jayakumar and Lalitha,[9] 2019:52)

My goal in writing this piece was to explain the politics between knowledge systems or how ontological domination may occur. One set of ideas are foisted upon others as a judge or guide, undermining them and their epistemic bases. It is not feasible for individual families who are already suffering to press for reform in such a system but accept what exists or else keep looking for something appropriate until they find it, if so. Therefore, it becomes the responsibility of both clinicians and legislators to understand and demand for greater autonomy for all systems, or allowances for their knowledge to operate freely, especially if they offer the scope for healing, recovery or cure, which biomedicine *does not.* Otherwise naming an existing institution a "mental health" specialty is yet another tokenism, to not be confused for what it obfuscates.

9 Jayakumar, M., Lalithaa, K.S. (2019). A clinical study on paranoid schizophrenia and its homeopathic management. *IOSR Journal of Dental and Medical Sciences.* Vol. 18, No. 5 Ser. 7: 52–56.

REFERENCES

Addlakha, R. (2008). *Deconstructing mental illness: An ethnography of psychiatry, women and the family.* Zubaan: New Delhi.

Aggarwal, N. (2008). Farmer suicides in India: The role of psychiatry and anthropology. *International Journal of Social Psychiatry.* Vol. 54: 291. DOI: 10.1177/0020764007088396

Ahearn, L.M. (2001). Language and agency. *Annual Review of Anthropology.* Vol. 30, No. 1: 109–137.

Alcoff, L.M. (2007). Mignolo's epistemology of coloniality. *CR: The New Centennial Review.* Vol. 7, No. 3: 79–101. ISSN 1532-687x.

Anderson, H. (1997). *Conversation, language and possibilities: A postmodern approach to therapy.* New York: Basic Books.

Anthony, W.A. (1993). Recovery from Mental Illness: The Guiding Vision of the Mental Health Service System in the 1990s. *Psychosocial Rehabilitation Journal*, 16, 11–23. Available at: https://doi.org/10.1037/h0095655.

Arbour, L. (2008). Arbour welcomes entry into force of "ground-breaking" convention on disabilities. Available at: https://www.un.org/development/desa/disabilities/arbour-welcomes-entry-into-force-of-ground-breaking-convention-on-disabilities.html.

Arstein-Kerslake, A., Gooding, P., Andrews, L. and McSherry, B. (2017). Human rights and unfitness to plead: The demands of the convention on the rights of persons with disabilities. *Human Rights Law Review.* Vol. 17: 399–419.

Asokan, T.V. (2015). WELCOME ADDRESS – PRESIDENT, *Indian Journal of Psychiatry.* Vol. 57, No. Suppl 1: S1–S2. Available at: https://journals.lww.com/indianjpsychiatry/Fulltext/2015/57001/WELCOME_ADDRESS___PRESIDENT.3.aspx

Banks, J. A. (1998). The lives and values of researchers: implications for educating citizens in a multicultural society. *Educational Researcher,* Vol. 27. No. 7: 4–17. https://doi.org/10.3102/0013189X027007004.

Banerjee, S. (2021). The doubted scientist and her vaccine revolution. *The Hindu,* 5th August. Available at: https://www.thehindu.com/opinion/op-ed/the-doubted-scientist-and-her-vaccine-revolution/article35732376.ece.

Barnes, C. and Mercer, G. (1997). Breaking the mould? An introduction to doing disability research. In Barnes, C. and Mercer, G. (eds.). *Doing disability research.* Leeds: The Disability Press: 1–14.

Barrable, A., Papadatou-Pastou, M. and Tzotzoli, P. (2018). Supporting mental health, wellbeing and study skills in higher education: An online intervention system. *International Journal of Mental Health System.* Vol. 12: 54. DOI: 10.1186/s13033-018-0233-z.

Barrett, A.E. (2000). Marital trajectories and mental health. *Journal of Health and Social Behaviour.* Vol. 41, No. 4: 451–464.

Bartlett, N. (2021). Welcoming spirits: Colonial development and the politics of affliction x recovering histories. Available at: August 20, 2021, from Somatosphere, http://somatosphere.net/forumpost/welcoming-spirits/.

Bathla, M., Singh, M. and Relan, P. (2016). Prevalence of anxiety and depressive symptoms among patients with hypothyroidism. *Indian Journal Endocrinology and Metabolism.* Vol. 20: 468–474.

Bayetti, C., Jadhav, S. and Deshpande, S.N. (2017). How do psychiatrists in India construct their professional identity? A critical literature review. *Indian Journal of Psychiatry.* Vol. 59, No. 1: 26–37.

Bayetti, C., Jadhav, S. and Jain, S. (2016). The re-covering self: A critique of the recovery-based approach in India's mental health care. *Disability & the Global South.* Vol. 3, No. 1: 889–909. Available at: https://disabilityglobalsouth.files.wordpress.com/2012/06/dgs-03-01-04.pdf

Beachum, L. (2010). The psychopathology of cinema: How mental illness and psychotherapy are portrayed in film. Grand Valley State University. *Honors Projects.* 56. Available at: http://scholarworks.gvsu.edu/honorsprojects/56.

Bener, A., Dafeeah, E.E. and Salem, M.O. (2013). A study of reasons of non-compliance of psychiatric treatment and patients' attitudes towards illness and treatment in Qatar. *Issues in Mental Health Nursing.* Vol. 34, No. 4: 273–280.

Benoit, L., Russo, T., Barry, C., Falissard, B. and Henckes, N. (2019). "You have to believe in something": Risk of psychosis and psychiatrists' beliefs in the self-fulfilling prophecy. *Social Science & Medicine,* Vol. 230: 20–29. DOI: 10.1016/j.socscimed.2019.03.035

Beresford, P. (2016). The role of survivor knowledge in creating alternatives to psychiatry. In Russo, J. and Sweeney, A. (eds.). *Searching for a rose garden: Challenging Psychiatry, fostering mad studies.* UK: PCCS Books.

Beresford, P. (2022). Introduction. In Beresford, P. and Russo, J. (eds.). *The Routledge international handbook of mad studies.* London and New York: Routledge: 1–16.

Beresford, P. and Russo, J. (2016). Supporting the sustainability of Mad studies and preventing its co-option. *Disability & Society.* DOI: 10.1080/09687599.2016.1145380

Besley, T. (A.C.) (2010). Governmentality of youth: Managing risky subjects. *Policy Futures in Education.* Vol. 8 No. 5: 528–547.

Bhambra, G.K. (2014). Postcolonial and decolonial dialogues. *Postcolonial Studies.* Vol. 17, No. 2: 115–121. DOI: 10.1080/13688790.2014.966414.

Bindhulakshmi, P. (2006). Women and mental illness: An ethnographic study in Kerala. Unpublished doctoral dissertation. Bombay: Indian Institute of Technology.

Bjornestad, J., Veseth, M., Davidson, L., Joa, I., Johannessen, J.O., Larsen, T.K., Melle, I. and Hegelstad, WtV. (2018). Psychotherapy in psychosis: Experiences of fully recovered service users. *Frontiers in Psychology.* Vol. 9, No. 1675: 1–7.

Borg, M. (2007). The Nature of recovery as lived in everyday life: Perspectives of individuals recovering from severe mental health problems. Unpublished Ph.D. thesis. Trondheim: Norwegian University of Science and Technology-NTNU.

Bossema, E.R., de Haar, C.A., Westerhuis, W., Beenackers, B.P., Blom, B.C., Appels, M.C. and van Oeveren, C.J. (2011). Psychoeducation for patients with a psychotic disorder: Effects on knowledge and coping. *Prim Care Companion CNS Disord*. Vol. 13, No. 4. DOI: 10.4088/PCC.10m01116

Boyle, M. (2007). The problem with diagnosis. *The Psychologist*. Vol. 20, No. 5: 290–292.

Bradley, B. and Ecks, S. (2018). Disentangling family life and hair pulling: Trichotillomania and relatedness. *Medical Anthropology*. DOI: 10.1080/01459740.2018.1476509.

Breakwell, G.M. (1993). Social representations and social identity. *Papers on Social Representations – Textes sur les Représentations Sociales*. Vol. 2, No. 3: 1–217.

Breggin, P.R. (2013). *Psychiatric drug withdrawal – A guide for prescribers, therapists, patients and their families*. New York: Springer Publishing Company.

Brewer, E. (2018). Coming out Mad, coming out disabled. In Donaldson, E.J. (ed.). *Literatures of madness: Disability studies and mental health*. New York: Palgrave, Macmillan: 11–30.

Bryne, L., Stratford, A. and Davidson, L. (2018). The global need for lived experience leadership. *Psychiatric Rehabilitation Journal*. Vol. 41, No. 1: 76–79. DOI: 10.1037/prj0000289

Bueter, A. (2019). Social epistemology and psychiatry. In R. Bluhm and S. Tekin (eds.). *Bloomsbury Companion to Philosophy of Psychiatry*. Bloomsbury: 485–503. DOI: 10.5040/9781350024090.ch-024

Burke, K. (1969). *A rhetoric of motives*. Berkeley and Los Angeles: University of California Press.

Burr, V. (2003). *Social constructionism*. London and New York: Routledge.

Burstow, B. (2013). A rose by any other name: Naming and the battle against psychiatry. In LeFrancois, B.A., Menzies, R. and Reaume, G. (eds.). *Mad matters: A critical reader in Canadian mad studies*, Toronto: Canadian Scholars' Press Inc.: 79–90.

Campbell, J. (2008). *The hero with a thousand faces*. Novalto: New World Library.

Campbell, L.A. and Kisely, S.R. (2009). Advance treatment directives for people with severe mental illness. *Cochrane Database System Review*. Jan; Vol. 21, No. 1: CD005963.

Carel, H. and Kidd, I.J. (2014). Epistemic injustice in healthcare: A philosophial analysis. *Medicine, Health Care and Philosophy*. Vol. 17, No. 4: 529–540.

Cassell, E.J. (1991). *The nature of suffering and the goals of medicine*. New York, Oxford: Oxford University Press.

Chamberlin, J. (1984). Speaking for ourselves: An overview of the ex-psychiatric inmates' movement. *Psychosocial Rehabilitation Journal*. Vol. VIII, No. 2, October: 56–62.

Chamberlin, J. (1998). Citizenship rights and psychiatric disability. *Psychiatric Rehabilitation Journal*. Vol. 2, No. 4: 405–408.

Clandinin, D.J. and Connelly, F.M. (2000). *Narrative inquiry: Experience and story in qualitative research*. San Francisco: Jossey-Bass.

Cohen, B.M.Z. (2008). *Mental health user narratives – new perspectives on illness and recovery.* New York: Palgrave Macmillan.

Cohen, B.M.Z. (2016). *Psychiatric hegemony: A Marxist theory of mental illness.* New Zealand: Palgrave Macmillan.

Cohen, C.I. (1993). The biomedicalization of psychiatry: A critical overview. *Community Mental Health Journal.* Vol. 29, No. 6: 509–521.

Costa, L. Voronka, J., Landry, D., McFarlane, B., Reville, D. and Church, K. (2012). Recovering our stories: A small act of resistance. *Studies in Social Justice,* Vol. 6, No. 1: 85–101.

Crean, M. (2018). Minority scholars and insider-outsider researcher status: Challenges along a personal, professional and political continuum [32 paragraphs]. *Forum Qualitative Sozialforschung / Forum: Qualitative Social Research.* Vol. 19, No. 1, Art. 17. DOI: 10.17169/fqs-19.1.2874.

Cummings, C.R. and Bentley, K.J. (2018). A recovery perspective on wellness: Connection, awareness, congruence. *Journal of Psychosocial Rehabilitation in Mental Health.* DOI: 10.1007/s40737-018-0118-0.

D'Arcy, M. (2019). "It tastes like order": Psychotic evidence for antipsychotic efficacy and medicated subjectivity. *ETHOS.* Vol. 47, No. 1: 89–107.

Dalal, P.K. (2019). Message from Vice President, Indian psychiatric society. *Indian Journal Psychiatry.* Vol. 61: S634.

Das, S., Doval, N., Mohammad, S., Dua, N. and Chatterjee, S.S. (2017). Psychiatry and cinema: What can we learn from the magical screen? *Shanghai Arch Psychiatry,* Oct 25; Vol. 29, No. 5: 310–313. Published online Oct 25. DOI: 10.11919/j.issn.1002-0829.217014.

Das, V. and Addlakha, R. (2001). Disability and domestic citizenship: Voice, gender, and the making of the subject. *Public Culture.* Vol. 13, No. 3: 511–531.

Davar, B.V. (2012). Gender and community mental health: Sharing experiences from our service program. In Chavan, B.S., Gupta, N., Arun, P. et al. (eds.). *Community mental health in India.* New Delhi: Jaypee: 136–147.

Davar, B.V. (2013). From Mental illness to disability: Choices for women users/survivors of psychiatry in self and identity constructions. In Addlakha, R. (ed.). *Disability studies in India: Global discourses, local realities.* New Delhi: Routledge: 333–362.

Davar, B.V. (2014). Globalizing psychiatry and the case of "vanishing" alternatives in a neo-colonial state. *Disability and the Global South.* Vol. 1, No. 2: 266–284.

Davar, B.V. (2015). Delivering justice, withdrawing care: The norms and etiquettes of "having" a mental illness. In Davar, B.V. and Ravindran, T.K.S. (eds.). *Gendering mental health: Knowledges, identities, and institutions.* New Delhi: Oxford University Press: 1–26.

Davar, B.V. and Lohokare, M. (2012). Recovering from psychosocial traumas – the place of dargahs in Maharashtra. In Sujatha, V. and Abraham, L. (eds.). *Medical pluralism in contemporary India.* New Delhi: Orient Blackswan Pvt Limited: 255–276.

Davidson, L. (2003). *Living outside mental illness: Qualitative studies of recovery in schizophrenia.* New York and London: New York University Press.

Davidson, L., Lawless, M.S. and Leary, F. (2005). Concepts of recovery: Competing or complementary? *Current Opinion in Psychiatry.* Vol. 18: 664–667.

Davidson, L., Rakfeldt, J. and Strauss, J. (2010). *The roots of the recovery movement in psychiatry-lessons learned.* Edinburgh: Wiley-Blackwell.

Davidson, L. and Roe, D. (2007). "Recovery from" and "recovery" in serious mental illness: One strategy for lessening confusion plaguing recovery. *Journal of Mental Health.* Vol. 16, No. 4: 459–470.

de Bhailís, C. and Flynn, E. (2017). Recognising legal capacity: Commentary and analysis of Article 12 CRPD. *International Journal of Law in Context.* Vol. 13, No. I: 6–21. DOI: 10.1017/S174455231600046X.

De Lissovoy, N. and Fregoso Bailon, R.O. (2019). Coloniality: Key dimensions and critical implications. In Ford, D. (ed.). *Keywords in radical philosophy and education: Common concepts for contemporary movements.* Koninklijke Brill NV, Leiden. DOI: 10.1163/9879004400467_007

Deegan, P.E. (1988). Recovery: The lived experience of rehabilitation. *Psychosocial Rehabilitation Journal.* Vol. 11, No. 4: 11.

Deegan, P.E. (1996). Recovery as a journey of the heart. *Psychiatric Rehabilitation Journal.* Vol. 19, No. 3: 91–97.

Degerman, D. (2020). Maladjusted to injustice? Political agency, medicalization, and the user/survivor movement, *Citizenship Studies.* DOI: 10.1080/13621025.2020.1745151

Dhanda, A. (2007). Legal capacity in the disability rights convention: Stranglehold of the past or lodestar for the future. *Syracuse Journal Int'l L & Com.* Vol. 34: 429–462.

Dhanda, A. (2016). For a rights-based approach. *Frontline,* September 16. Available at: https://frontline.thehindu.com/cover-story/for-a-rightsbased-approach/article9050228.ece#!

Dhanda, A. (2018). A disability studies reading of the law for persons with disabilities in India. In Ghai, A. (ed.). *Disability in South Asia: Knowledge and experience.* Los Angeles, London, New Delhi, Singapore, Washington DC, Melbourne: Sage: 383–400.

Dhanda, A. (2019). Legislating on mental health in India to achieve SDG3. In Davidson, L. (ed.). *The Routledge handbook of international development, mental health and wellbeing.* Abingdon and New York: Routledge: 373–384.

Diamond, S. (2012). Imagining possibilities outside the medicalization of humanity: A critical ethnography of a community trying to build a world free of sanism and psychiatric oppression. Ph.D. dissertation. Toronto: University of Toronto.

Dotson, K. (2011). Tracking epistemic violence, tracking practices of silencing. *Hypatia.* Vol. 26, No. 2: 236–257. DOI: 10.1111/j.1527-2001.2011.01177.x.

Dressler, W.W., Balieiro, M.C. and dos Santos, J.E. (2019). Agency, cultural consonance and depressive symptoms: A Brazilian Example. *Ethos.* Vol. 00: 1–20.

Duncombe, J. and Jessop, J. (2002). "Doing rapport" and the ethics of "faking friendship". In Mauthner, M., Birch, M., Jessop, J., and Miller, T. (eds.). *Ethics in qualitative research.* SAGE Publications Ltd: 108–122. DOI: 10.4135/9781849209090.

Fairclough, N. (1989/1996). *Language and power.* England: Addison Wesley Longman Limited.

Fairclough, N. (2003). *Analysing discourse-textual analysis for social research.* London and New York: Routledge.

Faugier, J. and Sargeant, M. (1997). Sampling hard to reach populations. *Journal of Advanced Nursing*. Vol. 26: 790–797.

Faulkner, A. (2004). *The ethics of survivor research: Guidelines for the ethical conduct of research carried out by mental health service users and survivors.* UK: The Policy Press.

Fee, D. (2000). The broken dialogue: mental illness as discourse and experience. In D. Fee (Ed.), *Pathology and the postmodern: Mental illness as discourse and experience*. SAGE Publications Ltd: 2–17, https://dx.doi.org/10.4135/9781446217252.n1

Firmin, R.L., Lysaker, P.H., Luther, L., Yanos, P.T., Leonhardt, B., Breier, A. and Vohs, J.L. (2018). Internalized stigma in adults with early phase versus prolonged psychosis. *Early Intervention in Psychiatry*. 1–7. DOI: 10.1111/eip.12553.

Foucault, M. (1982). Afterword: The subject and power. In H.L. Dreyfus and P. Rabinow (eds.). *Michel foucault: Beyond structuralism and hermeneutics*, 2nd edn. Brighton: The Harvester Press: 208–226.

Foucault, M. (2003). *The birth of the clinic: An archaeology of medical perception*. London: Routledge.

Frances, A. (2013). *Saving normal: An insider's revolt against out-of-control psychiatric diagnosis, DSM-5, Big Pharma, and the medicalization of ordinary life*. New York: William Morrow-Harper Collins.

Frank, A.W. (1997). *The wounded storyteller: Body, illness and ethics*. Chicago and London: The University of Chicago Press.

Fraser,N.(2000).Rethinkingrecognition.*NewLeftReview*.(II:3).Availableat:https://newleftreview.org/issues/II3/articles/nancy-fraser-rethinking-recognition. Accessed 27 February 2022.

Frass, M., Strassl, R. P., Friehs, H., Müllner, M., Kundi, M., & Kaye, A. D. (2012). Use and acceptance of complementary and alternative medicine among the general population and medical personnel: a systematic review. *The Ochsner Journal*, 12(1): 45–56.

Freire, P. (2000). *Pedagogy of the oppressed*. 30th anniversary ed. New York: Continuum.

Fricker, M. (2007). *Epistemic injustice: Power and the ethics of knowing*. New York: Oxford University Press.

Fricker, M. (2013). Epistemic justice as a condition of political freedom? *Synthese*. Vol. 190: 1317–1332.

Fullagar, S. (2017). Foucauldian theory, In Cohen, B. (ed.). *Routledge international handbook of critical mental health*. London: Routledge: 39–45.

Gammeltoft, T.M. and Oosterhoff, P. (2018). Mental health in domestic worlds. *Medical Anthropology*. Vol. 37, No. 7: 533–537.

Ganim, J.M. (2005). Identity and subjecthood. In Ellis, V. (ed.). *The Oxford student's guide to Chaucer*. Oxford: Oxford University Press: 224–238.

Gergen, K.J. (1985). The social constructionist movement in modern psychology. *American Psychologist*. Vol. 40, No. 3: 266–275.

Gergen, K.J. (1996). Social psychology as social construction: The emerging vision. In McGarty, C. and Haslam, A. (eds.). *The Message of social psychology: Perspectives on mind in society*. Oxford: Blackwell. Downloaded from: https://www.

swarthmore.edu/sites/default/files/assets/documents/kenneth-gergen/Social_Psychology_as_Social_Construction_The%20Emerging_Vision.pdf.

Gergen, K.J. (1997). *Realities and relationships: Soundings in social construction.* Massachusetts and London: Harvard University Press.

Gergen, K.J. (1998). Constructionism and realism: How are we to go on? In Parker, I. (ed.). *Social constructionism, discourse and realism.* London, Thousand Oaks, New Delhi: Sage Publications: 147–155.

Gergen, K.J. (1999). *An invitation to social construction.* London: Sage.

Gergen, K.J. (2001). *Social construction in context.* London, Thousand Oaks, New Delhi: Sage Publications.

Gergen, K.J. (2007). The self: Colonization in psychology and society. *Psychology's Territories: Historical and Contemporary Perspectives from Different Disciplines.* 149–167. https://works.swarthmore.edu/fac-psychology/600

Gergen, K.J. (2009). *An invitation to social construction.* Los Angeles, London, New Delhi, Singapore, Washington DC: Sage.

Gergen, K.J. (2014). From mirroring to world-making: Research as future forming. *Journal for the Theory of Social Behaviour.* DOI: 10.1111/jtsb.12075

Gergen, K.J. and Gergen, M.M. (2008). *Social construction: Entering the dialogue.* Ohio: Taos Institute Publications.

Gergen, K.J. and Gergen, M.M. (2011). Narrative tensions: Perilous and productive. *Narrative Inquiry.* Vol. 21, No. 2: 374–381.

Ghosh, N. (2018). Experiencing the body: Feminity, sexuality and disabled women in India. In Ghai, A. (ed.). *Disability in South Asia: Knowledge and experience.* Los Angeles, London, New Delhi, Singapore, Washington DC, Melbourne: Sage.

Goffman, E. (1961/1991). *Asylums: Essays on the social situation of mental patients and other inmates.* United Kingdom: Penguin Books.

Goffman, E. (1963). *Stigma-notes on the management of a spoiled identity.* New York, London, Toronto: Simon and Schuster, Inc.

Gonzalez Casanova, P. (1965). Internal colonialism and national development. *Studies in Comparative International Development.* Vol. 1, No. 4: 27–37. DOI: 10.1007/bf02800542

Gøtzsche, P.C. (2015). *Deadly psychiatry and organised denial.* Denmark: People's Press.

Greenberg, J.S., Kim, H.W. and Greenley, J.R. (1997). Factors associated with subjective burden in siblings of adults with severe mental illness. *American Journal of Orthopsychiatry.* Vol. 67, No. 2: 231–241.

Gyan, P. (1995). Introduction: After colonialism. In Gyan, P. (ed.). *After colonialism: Imperial histories and postcolonial displacements.* Princeton, NJ: Princeton University Press: 3–17.

Hacking, I. (1999). *The social construction of what?* England, MA: Harvard University Press.

Haider, A. (2018). How cinema stigmatizes mental illness. Available at: http://www.bbc.com/culture/story/20180828-how-cinema-stigmatises-mental-illness.

Halliburton, M. (2004). Finding a fit: Psychiatric pluralism in South India and its implications for who studies of mental disorder. *Transcultural Psychiatry.* Vol. 41, No. 1: 80–98.

Hanley, E. (2015). Perception of mental illness based upon its portrayal in film. University of Central Florida. Available at: https://stars.library.ucf.edu/honorstheses1990-2015/609.

Harper, D. and Speed, E. (2012). Uncovering recovery: The resistible rise of recovery and resilience. *Studies in Social Justice*. Vol. 6, No. 1: 9–25.

Harper, D.J. (2013). On the persistence of psychiatric diagnosis: Moving beyond a zombie classification system. *Feminism & Psychology*. Vol. 23, No. 1: 78–85.

Healy, D. (2006). The latest mania: Selling bipolar disorder. *PLoS Med*. Vol. 3, No. 4: e185.

Healy, D. (2012). *Pharmageddon*. Los Angeles: University of California Press.

Helman, D.S. (2017). Recovery from Schizophrenia: An autoethnography, *Deviant Behavior*: 1–20. DOI: http://www.tandfonline.com/doi/abs/10.1080/01639625.2017.1286174

Herrman, H. and Swartz, L. (2007). Promotion of mental health in poorly resourced countries. *The Lancet*. Vol. 370, October 6. DOI: 10.1016/S0140-6736(07)61244-6

Hiruy, K. (2014). Using multi-sited ethnographic case studies and auto-ethnography to explore bottom-up community empowerment among African communities in Australia. In *Sage Research Methods*. DOI: 10.4135/9781446274305014537443.

Holborow, M. (2007). Language, ideology and neoliberalism. *Journal of Language and Politics*. Vol. 6, No. 1: 51–73.

Holmes, A.G.D. (2020). Researcher positionality – a consideration of its influence and place in qualitative research – a new researcher guide. *Shanlax International Journal of Education*. Vol. 8, No. 4: 1–10. DOI: 10.34293/education.v8i4.3232

Hyden, L.-C. (1997). Illness and narrative. *Sociology of Health and Illness*. Vol. 19, No. 1: 48–69.

Ingleby, D. (1980). Understanding "mental illness". In Ingleby, D. (ed.). *Critical psychiatry – The politics of mental health*. New York: Pantheon Books: 23–71.

Ingram, R.A. (2008). "Mapping 'Mad studies': The birth of an in/discipline". Disability Studies Student Conference, Syracuse University. New York: Syracuse.

Ivbijaro, G. (2012). The case of change: The global mental health action plan 2013–2020. *Mental Health in Family Medicine*. Vol. 9: 135. Available at: https://www.ncbi.nlm.nih.gov/pmc/articles/PMC3622905/pdf/MHFM-09-135.pdf.

Jacob, K.S. (2015). Recovery model of mental illness: A complementary approach to psychiatric care. *Indian Journal Psychology Medicine*. Vol. 37, No. 2: 117–119.

Janks, H. (1997). Critical discourse analysis as a research tool. *Discourse: Studies in the Cultural Politics of Education*. Vol. 18, No. 3: 329–334.

Jara, R.S. and Pisani, A.M.O. (2020). New and old knowledge aimed at decolonising mental health: Reflections and proposals from Chile. *International Review of Psychiatry*. Vol. 32, No. 4: 334–339. DOI: 10.1080/09540261.2020.1767042

Jarman, J. (2001). Explaining social exclusion. *International Journal of Sociology and Social Policy*. Vol. 21, No. 4/5/6: 3–9. DOI: 10.1108/01443330110789411.

Jasanoff, S. (ed.) (2011). *Reframing rights. Bioconstitutionalism in the genetic age*. Cambridge MA: MIT Press.

Johnston, M.S. (2019). Stories of madness: Exploring resistance, conformity, resiliency, agency, and disengagement in mental health narratives. Unpublished doctoral dissertation. Ottawa: Carleton University.

Jones, N., Shattell, M., Kelly, T., Brown, R., Robinson, L., Renfro, R., Harris, B. and Luhrmann, T.M. (2016). "Did I push myself over the edge?": Complications of agency in psychosis onset and development. *Psychosis.* DOI: 10.1080/17522439.2016.1150501.

Jorm, A.F. (2000). Mental health literacy: Public knowledge and beliefs about mental disorders. *British Journal of Psychiatry.* Vol. 177: 396–401.

Joseph, A.J. (2019). Constituting "lived experience" discourses in mental health: The ethics of racialized identification/representation and the erasure of intergeneration colonial violence. *Journal of Ethics in Mental Health.* Open Volume: 1–23.

Jovchelovitch, S. (2008). Reflections on the diversity of knowledge: Power and dialogue in representational fields. In Sugiman, T., Gergen, K.J., Wagner, W. and Yamada, Y. (eds.). *Meaning in action: Constructions, narratives and representations.* Japan: Springer: 23–36.

Jungbauer, J., Wittmund, B., Dietrich, S. and Angermeyer, M.C. (2004). The disregarded caregivers: Subjective burden in spouses of schizophrenia patients. *Schizophrenia Bulletin.* Vol. 30, No. 3: 665–675.

Jutel, A. (2017). "The expertness of his healer": Diagnosis, disclosure and the power of a profession. *Health*: 1–17. DOI: 10.1177/1363459317745956.

Kala, A.K. (2012). Covert medication in psychiatry: A case for taking it out of the closet and using it rationally, without being apologetic. *Indian Journal of Psychiatry.* Vol. 54, No. 3: 257–265.

Kamble, M.T., Nandedkar, P.D., Dharme, P.V., Lohkhande, S.L. and Bhosale, P.G. (2013). Thyroid function and mental disorders: An insight into the complex interaction. *Journal of Clinical and Diagnostic Research.* Vol. 7, No. 1: 11–14.

Kaur, R. and Pathak, R.K. (2017). Treatment gap in mental healthcare: Reflections from policy and research. *Economic and Political Weekly.* Vol. LII, No. 31: August 5.

Kiossev, A. (1995). Notes on self-colonising cultures. *Cultural Aspects of the Modernisation Process.* Oslo.

Kiossev, A. The self-colonizing metaphor. Published electronically in the Atlas of transformation. Available at: http://monumenttotransformation.org/atlas-of-transformation/html/s/self-colonization/the-self-colonizing-metaphor-alexander-kiossev.html

Kirk, S.A., Gomory, T. and Cohen, D. (2013). *Mad Science: Psychiatric coercion, diagnosis, and drugs.* USA and UK: Transaction Publishers.

Kuhn, T.S. (1962). *The structure of scientific revolutions.* Chicago: University of Chicago Press.

Kulhara, P., Chakrabarti, S., Avasthi, A., Sharma, A. and Sharma, S. (2009). Psychoeducational intervention for caregivers of Indian patients with schizophrenia: A randomised-controlled trial. *Acta Psychiatrica Scandinavica.* Vol. 119, No. 6: 472–483.

Kulkarni, V.S. and Gaiha, R. (2017). Mind the treatment gap – Implementation of the mental healthcare act will require a restructuring of health-care services. *The Hindu*, April, 11.

Kumar, M.T. (2018). Mental healthcare Act 2017: Liberal in principles, let down in provisions. *Indian Journal Psychology Medicine.* Vol. 40: 101–107.

Kvale, S. (2006). Dominance through interviews and dialogues. *Qualitative Inquiry*. Vol. 12, No. 3: 480–500.

Larsan-Barr, M. (2016). Experiencing antipsychotic medication: From first prescriptions to attempted discontinuation. Unpublished doctoral dissertation. New Zealand: University of Auckland.

Lather, P. (1986). Research as praxis. *Harvard Educational Review*. Vol. 56, No. 3: 257–277.

Law, H. (2014). Understanding recovery in psychosis. Unpublished doctoral dissertation. United Kingdom: University of Manchester.

Leavy, P. (2014). Introduction. In Leavy, P. (ed.). *The Oxford handbook of qualitative research*. New York: Oxford University Press: 1–13.

Lee, J-E., (2013). Mad as hell: The objectifying experience of symbolic violence. In LeFrancois, B.A., Menzies, R., Reaume, G. (eds.). *Mad matters: A critical reader in Canadian mad studies*. Toronto: Canadian Scholars' Press Inc.: 105–121.

LeFrancois, B.A., Menzies, R. and Reaume, G. (Eds.) (2013). *Mad matters: A critical reader in Canadian mad studies*. Toronto: Canadian Scholars' Press Inc.

Lemke, T. (2002). Foucault, governmentality, and critique. *Rethinking Marxism*. Vol. 14, No. 3: 49–64. DOI: 10.1080/089356902101242288

Liberman, R.P. and Kopelowicz, A. (2005). Recovery from schizophrenia: A concept in search of research. *Psychiatric Services*. Vol. 56, No. 6: 735–742.

Liegghio, M. (2013). A denial of being: Psychiatrization as epistemic violence. In LeFrancois, B.A., Menzies, R. and Reaume, G. (eds.). *Mad matters: A critical reader in Canadian mad studies*. Toronto: Canadian Scholars' Press Inc.: 122–129.

Link, B.G. and Phelan, J.C. (2001). Conceptualizing stigma. *Annual Review of Sociology*. Vol. 27: 363–385.

Link, B.G., Rahav, M., Phelan, J.C. and Nuttbrock, L. (1997). On stigma and its consequences: Evidences from a longitudinal study of men with dual diagnoses of mental illness and substance abuse. *Journal of Health and Social Behaviour*. Vol. 38 (June): 177–190.

Llewellyn-Beardsley, J., Rennick-Egglestone, S., Callard, F., Crawford, P., Farkas, M., Hui, A., et al. (2019). Characteristics of mental health recovery narratives: Systematic review and narrative synthesis. *PLoS ONE*. Vol. 14, No. 3: e0214678. DOI: 10.1371/journal.pone.0214678

Locke, J. (1690/ 2012). Second treatise of government. Available at: https://english.hku.hk/staff/kjohnson/PDF/LockeJohnSECONDTREATISE1690.pdf.

Luhrmann, T.M. (2016). Introduction. In Luhrmann, T.M. and Marrow, J. (eds.). *Our most troubling madness: Case studies in schizophrenia across cultures*. California: University of California Press: 1–25.

Luhrmann, T.M. and Padmavati, R. (2016). Voices that are more benign – the experience of auditory hallucinations in Chennai. In Luhrmann, T.M. and Marrow, J. (eds.). *Our most troubling madness: Case studies in schizophrenia across cultures*. California: University of California Press: 99–112.

Lysaker, P.H., Taylor, A., Miller, A., Beattie, N., Strasburger, A. and Davis, L.W. (2006). The scale to assess narrative development. *The Journal of Nervous and Mental Disease*. Vol. 194, No. 3: 223–225.

215

MacGregor, H. (2018). Mental Health and the Maintenance of Kinship in South Africa. *Medical Anthropology*. DOI: 10.1080/01459740.2018.1508211.

Machin, D. and Mayr, A. (2012). *How to do critical discourse analysis: A multimodal introduction*. Los Angeles, London, New Delhi, Singapore, Washington DC: Sage.

Mann, C.E. and Himelein, M.J. (2004). Factors associated with stigmatization of persons with mental illness. *Psychiatric Services*. Vol. 55, No. 2: 185–187. DOI: 10.1176/appi.ps.55.2.185.

Manohar, N., Liamputtong, P., Bhole, S. and Arora, A. (2017). Researcher positionality in cross cultural and sensitive research. In P. Liamputtong (ed.). *Handbook of research methods in health social sciences*, Springer Nature Singapore Pte Ltd. DOI: 10.1007/978-981-10-2779-6_35-1

Marrow, J. (2016). Vulnerable transitions in a World of Kin: In the shadow of good wifeliness in North India. In Luhrmann, T.M. and Marrow, J. (eds.). *Our most troubling madness: Case studies in schizophrenia across cultures*. California: University of California Press: 56–70.

Marrow, J. and Luhrmann, T.M. (2016). Conclusion. In Luhrmann, T.M. and Marrow, J. (eds.). *Our most troubling madness: Case studies in schizophrenia across cultures*. California: University of California Press: 197–222.

Mathias, K. (2016). Shadow and light: Examining community mental health competence in North India. Department of Public Health and Clinical Medicine Epidemiology and Global Health. Unpublished doctoral thesis. Sweden: Umea University.

Mathias, K., Kermode, M., Goicolea, I., Seefeldt, L., Shidhaye, R. and San Sebastian, M. (2018). Social distance and community attitudes towards people with psycho-social disabilities in Uttarakhand, India. *Community Mental Health Journal*. Vol. 54: 343–353.

Mathias, K., Kermode, M., San Sebastian, M., Davar, B. and Goicolea, I. (2018). An asymmetric burden: Experiences of men and women as caregivers of people with psycho-social disabilities in rural North India. *Transcultural Psychiatry*. Vol. 0, No. 0: 1–27. DOI: 10.1177/1363461518792728

Mathias, K., Kermode, M., San Sebastian, M., Koschorke, M. and Goicolea, I. (2015). Under the banyan tree – Exclusion and inclusion of people with mental disorders in rural North India. *BMC Public Health*. Vol. 15: 446.

Maulik, P.K., Devarapalli, S., Kallakuri, S., Tewari, A., Chilappagari, S., Koschorke, M. and Thornicroft, G. (2017). Evaluation of an anti-stigma campaign related to common mental disorders in rural India: A mixed methods approach. *Psychological Medicine*. Vol. 47, No. 3: 565–575. DOI: 10.1017/S0033291716002804.

Mazza, G. (2016). Work and respect in Chennai. In Luhrmann, T.M. and Marrow, J. (eds.). *Our most troubling madness – Case studies in schizophrenia across cultures*. California: University of California Press: 71–85.

McNamee, S. (1989). Challenging the patriarchal vision of social science: Lessons from a family therapy model. In Carter, K. and Spitzack, C. (eds.). *Doing research on women's communication: Perspectives on theory and method*. New Jersey: Ablex Publishing Corporation: 95–117.

Medina, J. (2011). The relevance of credibility excess in a proportional view of epistemic injustice: Differential epistemic authority and the social imaginary,

Social Epistemology: A Journal of Knowledge, Culture and Policy. Vol. 25, No. 1: 15–35.

Mellor, J., Ingram, N., Abrahams, J. and Beedell, P. (2014). Class matters in the interview setting? Positionality, situatedness and class. *The British Educational Research Journal.* Vol. 40, No. 1: 135–149.

Menzies, R., LeFrancois, B.A. and Reaume, G. (2013). Introducing mad studies. In LeFrancois, B.A., Menzies, R., Reaume, G. (eds.). *Mad matters: A critical reader in Canadian mad studies,* Toronto: Canadian Scholars' Press Inc.: 1–22.

Merrell, W.C. and Shalts, E. (2002). Homeopathy. *Medical Clinics of North America.* Vol. 86, No. 1: 47–62. DOI: 10.1016/s0025-7125(03)00071-3.

Merriam, S.B., Johnson-Bailey, J., Lee, M.-Y., Kee, Y., Ntseane, G. and Muhamad, M. (2001). Power and positionality: Negotiating insider/outsider status within and across cultures. *International Journal of Lifelong Education.* Vol. 20, No. 5: 405–416.

Mignolo, W.D. (2009). Epistemic disobedience, independent thought and decolonial freedom. *Theory, Culture & Society.* Vol. 26, No. (7–8): 1–23. DOI: 10.1177/0263276409349275

Miller, L. (2008). A personal perspective on recovery. *Chronic Illness.* Vol. 4: 311.

Mills, C. (2014). *Decolonizing global mental health: The psychiatrization of the majority world.* London and New York: Routledge.

Mills, C. and Hilberg, E. (2020). The construction of mental health as a technological problem in India. *Critical Public Health.* Vol. 30, No. 1: 41–52. DOI: 10.1080/09581596.2018.1508823

Ministry of Health and Family Welfare (2013). The Mental health Care Bill 2013. Available at: https://prsindia.org/billtrack/the-mental-health-care-bill-2013#:~:text=The%20Mental%20Health%20Care%20Bill%2C%202013%20was%20introduced%20in%20the, Persons%20with%20Disabilities%20in%20 2007, accessed on 27th February 2022.

Ministry of Health and Family Welfare (2014). National Mental Health Policy of India: New Pathways, New Hope. Available at: https://nhm.gov.in/images/pdf/National_Health_Mental_Policy.pdf, accessed on 27th February 2022.

Moncrieff, J. (2013). *The bitterest pills: The troubling story of antipsychotic drugs.* London: Palgrave Macmillan.

Morrison, L.J. (2008). *Talking back to psychiatry: The psychiatric consumer/survivor/ex-patient movement.* New York & London: Routledge.

Morrow, M. and Weisser, J. (2012). Towards a social justice framework of mental health recovery. *Studies in Social Justice.* Vol. 6, No. 1: 27–43.

Morrow, V. (2001). Young people's explanations and experiences of social exclusion: Retrieving Bourdieu's concept of social capital. *International Journal of Sociology and Social Policy.* Vol. 21, No. 4/5/6: 37–63.

Murthy, S.R. (2011). Mental health initiatives in India (1947–2010). *The National Medical Journal of India.* Vol. 24, No. 2: 98–107.

Myers, N.A.L. (2016). Recovery stories: An anthropological exploration of moral agency in stories of mental health recovery. *Transcultural Psychiatry.* Vol. 53, No. 4: 427–444.

Myers, N.A.L. and Ziv, T. (2016). "No one ever even asked me that before": Autobiographical power, social defeat, and recovery among African Americans with lived experiences of psychosis. *Medical Anthropology Quarterly*. Vol. 30, No. 3: 395–413.

Nagaraj, V. (2015). Adjudicating illness and capacity: Notes from a custody trial. In Davar, B.V., and Ravindran, T.K.S. (eds.). *Gendering mental health: Knowledges, identities and institutions*. New Delhi: Oxford University Press: 51–70.

Nandy, A. (2009). *The intimate enemy: Loss and recovery of self under colonialism*. Delhi: Oxford University Press.

Nunley, M. (1996). Why psychiatrists in India prescribe so many drugs. *Culture, Medicine and Psychiatry*. Vol. 20: 165–197.

Nunley, M. (1998). The involvement of families in Indian psychiatry. *Culture, Medicine and Psychiatry*. Vol. 22, No. 3: 317–353.

O'Donnell, A., Sapouna, L. and Brosnan, L. (2019). Storytelling: An act of resistance or a commodity? *Journal of Ethics in Mental Health*. Open Volume: 1–13.

Oliver, M. (1990). *The politics of disablement*. London: Macmillan.

Oliver, M. (1992). Changing the social relations of research production? *Disability, Handicap & Society*. Vol. 7, No. 2: 101–114.

Ortner, S.B. (2006). *Anthropology and social theory: Culture, power and the acting subject*. Durham and London: Duke University Press.

Parker, I. (2005). *Qualitative psychology: Introducing radical research*. England: Open University Press.

Parkinson, H.J. (2018). Unsane: How film's portrayal of mental illness is (slowly) improving. *The Guardian*. 23rd March. Available at: https://www.theguardian.com/film/2018/mar/23/unsane-a-history-of-mental-illness-in-film.

Pasquini, M.W. and Olaniyan, O. (2004). The researcher and the field assistant: A cross-disciplinary, cross-cultural viewing of positionality. *Interdisciplinary Science Reviews*. Vol. 29, No. 1: 24–36.

Pathare, S., Kalha, J. and Krishnamoorthy, S. (2018). Peer support for mental illness in India: An underutilized resource. *Epidemiology and Psychiatric Sciences*. Cambridge University Press. DOI: 10.1017/S2045796018000161.

Pattadath, B. (2016). Experience as "expert" knowledge: A critical understanding of survivor research in mental health. *Philosophy, Psychiatry, & Psychology*. Vol. 23, No. 3/4: 203–205.

Pescosolido, B.A., Martin, J.K., Long, J.S., Medina, T.R., Phelan, J.C. and Link, B.G. (2010). "A disease like any other"? A decade of change in public reactions to schizophrenia, depression, and alcohol dependence. *The American Journal of Psychiatry*. Vol. 167: 1321–1330.

Philip, S., Rangarajan, S.K., Moirangthem, S., Kumar, C.N., Gowda, M.R., Gowda, G.S., et al. (2019). Advance directives and nominated representatives: A critique. *Indian Journal Psychiatry*. Vol. 61: S680–S685.

Pilgrim, D. (2008). "Recovery" and current mental health policy. *Chronic Illness*. Vol. 4: 295–304.

Pinto, S. (2013). Movement in time: Choreographies of confinement in an inpatient ward. In Trnka, S., Dureau, C. and Park, J. (eds.). *Senses and citizenship: Embodying political life*. New York: Routledge: 79–98.

Pirkis, J., Blood, R.W., Francis, C. and McCallum, K. (2006). On-screen portrayals of mental illness: Extent, nature, and impacts. *Journal of Health Communication*. Vol. 11, No. 5: 523–541. DOI: 10.1080/10810730600755889.

Pitschel-Walz, G., Bäuml, J., Bender, W., Engel, R.R., Wagner, M. and Kissling, W. (2006). Psychoeducation and compliance in the treatment of schizophrenia: Results of the Munich Psychosis Information project study. *The Journal of Clinical Psychiatry.* Mar; Vol. 67, No. 3: 443–452. DOI: 10.4088/jcp.v67n0316

Pohlhaus, G. Jr. (2014). Discerning the primary epistemic harm in cases of testimonial injustice. *Social Epistemology.* Vol. 28, No. 2: 99–114. DOI: 10.1080/02691728.2013.782581

polanco, m. and X, Tisha (2021). Andean decoloniality and mental health. In Lester, J.N. and O'Reilly, M. (eds.). *The Palgrave encyclopedia of critical perspectives on mental health,*

Pompili, M., Harnic, D., Gonda, X., Forte, A., Dominici, G., Innamorati, M., Fountoulakis, K.N., Serafini, G., Sher, L., Janiri, L., Rihmer, Z., Amore, M., and Girardi, P. (2014). Impact of living with bipolar patients: Making sense of caregivers' burden. *World Journal Psychiatry.* Vol. 4, No. 1: 1–12.

Porter, M. (2015). Colonization by/in psychiatry: From over-medicalization to democratization. *Journal of Ethics in Mental Health.* Open Volume 1: 1–7.

Potter, N.N. (2015). Colonizing forces in psychiatry. *Journal of Ethics in Mental Health.* Open Volume 1: 1.

Priya, R. and Ghodajkar, P. (2018). The structural basis of corruption in healthcare in India. In Nundy, S., Desiraju, K. and Nagral, S. (eds.). *Healers or predators? Healthcare corruption in India.* New Delhi: Oxford University Press: 3–43.

Puras, D. and Gooding, P. (2019). Mental health and human rights in the 21st century. *World Psychiatry.* Vol. 18, No. 1: 42–43.

Rakhshan, M., Ghanbari, A.R., Rahimi, A. and Mostafavi, I. (2017). A Comparison between the quality of life and mental health of patients with hypothyroidism and normal people referred to Motahari clinic of Shiraz University of medical sciences. *International Journal of Community Based Nursing and Midwifery.* Vol. 5, No. 1: 30–37.

Ranganathan, S. (2011). Making sense of suffering: Spirit possession in Mahanubhav temples in Maharashtra, India. Unpublished doctoral dissertation. Bombay: Indian Institute of Technology.

Rebughini, P. (2015). Subject, subjectivity, subjectivation between autonomy and ethics: Reply to the commentaries. *Sociopedia.isa.* DOI: 10.1177/20568460027.

Reddy, V.B., Gupta, A., Lohiya, A. and Kharya, P. (2013). Mental health issues and challenges in India: A review. *International Journal of Scientific and Research Publications.* Vol. 3, No. 2: 1–3.

Reynolds, J.F. (2018). A short history of mental health rhetoric research (MHRR). *Rhetoric of Health and Medicine.* Vol. 1, No. 1–2: 1–18.

Richardson, E.T. (2020). *Epidemic illusions: on the coloniality of global public health.* Cambridge, MA and England: The MIT Press.

Rimke, H. (2018). Sickening institutions: A feminist sociological analysis and critique of religion, medicine, and psychiatry. In Kilty, J. and Dej, E. (eds.). *Containing madness.* Palgrave Macmillan, Cham. DOI: 10.1007/978-3-319-89749-3_2.

Roberts, G. and Boardman, J. (2013). Understanding "recovery". *Advances in Psychiatric Treatment.* Vol. 19: 400–409.

Roberts, M. (2005). The production of psychiatric subject: Power, knowledge and Michel Foucault. *Nursing Philosophy.* Vol. 6: 33–42.

Roe, D. and Lachman, M. (2005). The subjective experience of people with severe mental illness: A potentially crucial piece of the puzzle. *The Israel Journal of Psychiatry and Related Sciences*, Vol. 42, No. 4: 223–230.

Roe, D., Mashiach-Eizenberg, M. and Lysaker, P.H. (2011). The relation between objective and subjective domains of recovery among persons with schizophrenia-related disorders. *Schizophrenia Research.* Vol. 131: 133–138.

Rogers, A. and Pilgrim, D. (2005). *A sociology of mental health and illness.* England: Open University Press.

Rorty, R.M. (1992). Introduction: Metaphilosophical difficulties of linguistic philosophy. In Rorty, R.M. (ed.). *The linguistic turn: Essays in philosophical method.* Chicago and London: The University of Chicago Press: 1–39.

Rose, D. (2019). Navigating an insider/outsider identity in exclusive academic spaces: How far can boundaries be pushed? *Journal of Ethics in Mental Health.* Open Vol. 10: 1–18.

Rosenhan, D.L. (1973). On being sane in insane places. *Science.* Vol. 179, No. 70: 250–258.

Roy, R., Jahan, M., Kumari, S. and Chakraborty, P.K. (2005). Reasons for drug non-compliance of psychiatric patients: A centre based study. *Journal of the Indian Academy of Applied Psychology.* Vol. 31, No. 1–2: 24–28.

Russo, J. (2016). Towards our own framework, or reclaiming madness part two. In Russo, J. and Sweeney, A. (eds.). *Searching for a rose garden: Challenging Psychiatry, fostering mad studies.* UK: PCCS Books: 59–68.

Russo, J. (2019). Unmaking madness: Exploring collective first-person epistemology. Unpublished doctoral dissertation. London: Brunel University.

Russo, J. and Beresford, P. (2015). Between exclusion and colonisation: Seeking a place for mad people's knowledge in academia. *Disability & Society.* Vol. 30, No. 1: 153–157. DOI: 10.1080/09687599.2014.957925

Russo, J. and Wallcraft, J. (2011). Resisting variables: Service user/survivor perspectives on researching coercion. In Kallert, T.W., Mezzich, J.E., Monahan, J. (eds.). *Coercive treatment in psychiatry: Clinical, legal and ethical aspects.* John Wiley & Sons Ltd: 213–234.

Saldana, J. (2011). *Fundamentals of qualitative research.* New York: Oxford University Press.

Sarin, A. (2012). On covert medication: The issues involved. *Indian Journal of Psychiatry.* Vol. 54: 271–272.

Sarin, A. and Jain, S. (2017). Mapping difficult terrains: The writing of policy on mental health. In White, R.G. et al. (eds.). *The palgrave handbook of sociocultural perspectives on global mental health.* DOI: 10.1057/978-1-137-39510-8_33.

Sarin, A., Murthy, P. and Chatterjee, S. (2012). Psychiatric advance directives: Potential challenges in India. *Indian Journal of Medical Ethics.* Vol. IX, No. 2 April–June: 104–107.

Savin-Baden, M. and Major, C.H. (2013). *Qualitative research: The essential guide to theory and practice.* Abingdon: Routledge.

Scheff, T.J. (1999). *Being mentally ill: A sociological theory.* New York: Aldine De Gruyter.

Scott, J.W. (1991). The evidence of experience. *Critical Inquiry.* Vol. 17, No. 4: 773–797.

Scott, S. and Geddes, A. (2016). Ethics, methods and moving standards in research on migrant workers and forced labour. In D. Siegel, R. de Wildt (eds.). *Ethical concerns in research on human trafficking*, Studies of Organized Crime 13, DOI: 10.1007/978-3-319-21521-1_8. Springer International Publishing.

Sewell, WH. Jr. (1992). A theory of structure: Duality, agency, and transformation. *American Journal of Sociology.* Vol. 98, No. 1: 1–29.

Shakespeare, T. (2018). *Disability: The basics.* London and New York: Routledge.

Sharma, P. (2011). Mending the broken frame: Self narration in a constructionist framework. *Psychological Studies.* Vol. 57, No. 2: 189–194.

Sharma, P. (2014). Making song, making sanity: Recovery from bipolar disorder. *Canadian Journal of Music Therapy.* Vol. 20, No. 1: 65–84.

Sharma, P. (2015). Musical progressions: A multimodal approach in healing from bipolar disorder. *World Cultural Psychiatry Research Review.* September/October: 285–297.

Sharma, P. (2019). Peer support in mental healthcare. *Economic and Political Weekly.* Vol. 54, Nos. 26 & 27: 27–29.

Sharma, P. (2019a). The mental health imbroglio: to treat or to heal? *Economic and Political Weekly.* Vol. 54, No. 17: 12–14.

Sharma, V., Holmes, J.H. and Sarkar, I.N. (2016). Identifying complementary and alternative medicine usage information from internet resources: A systematic review. *Methods of Information in Medicine.* August 5; Vol. 55, No. 4: 322–332.

Shields-Zeeman, L., Pathare, S., Walters, B.H., Kapadia-Kundu, N. and Joag, K. (2017). Promoting wellbeing and improving access to mental health care through community champions in rural India: The Atmiyata intervention approach. *International Journal of Mental Health Systems.* Vol. 11, No. 6. DOI 10.1186/s13033-016-0113-3.

Sholl, J. (2017). The muddle of medicalization: Pathologizing or medicalizing? *Theoretical Medicine and Bioethics.* Vol. 38: 265–278.

Shotter, J. (2016). Ontological risks and communication anxieties: On what and whom others will "allow" us to be. *International Journal of Collaborative Practice.* Vol. 6, No. 1: 1–12.

Simpson, T. (2016). The sunrise project: Helping adults recover from psychiatric drugs. In Russo, J. and Sweeney, A. (eds.). *Searching for a rose garden: Challenging Psychiatry, fostering mad studies.* UK: PCCS Books: 152–159.

Slade, M. (2010). Mental illness and well-being: The central importance of positive psychology and recovery approaches. *BMC Health Services Research.* Vol. 10, No. 26. Downloaded from http://www.biomedcentral.com/1472–6963/10/26.

Slade, M. and Hayward, M. (2007). Recovery, psychosis and psychiatry: Research is better than rhetoric. *Acta Psychiatrica Scandinavica.* Vol. 116, No. 2: 81–83. DOI: 10.1111/j.1600-0447.2007.01047.x.

Slade, M., Amering, M. and Oades, L. (2008). Recovery: An international perspective. *Epidemiologia e Psichiatria Sociale.* Vol. 17: 128–137.

Smith, V., Reddy, J., Foster, K., Asbury, E.T. and Brooks, J. (2011). Public perceptions, knowledge and stigma towards people with schizophrenia. *Journal of Public Mental Health.* Vol. 10, No. 1: 45–56.

Sommer, M., Biong, S., Borg, M., Karlsson, B., Klevan, T., Ness, O., Nesse, L., Oute, J., Sundet, R. and Kim, H.S. (2021). Part II: Living life: A meta-synthesis exploring recovery as processual experiences. *International Journal of Environmental Research and Public Health.* Vol. 18: 6115. DOI: 10.3390/ijerph18116115

Sommer, R. (2011). The etymology of psychosis. *The American Journal of Orthopsychiatry*, Vol. 81, No. 2: 162–166. DOI: 10.1111/j.1939-0025.2011.01084.x.

Sood, A. (2015). Women's rights, human rights, and the State: Reconfiguring gender and mental health concerns in India. In Davar, B.V. and Ravindran, T.K.S. (eds.). *Gendering mental health: Knowledges, identities and institutions.* New Delhi: Oxford University Press: 162–192.

Sood, A. (2016). Madness experienced as faith: Temple healing in North India. In Luhrmann, T.M. and Marrow, J. (eds.). *Our most troubling madness: Case studies in schizophrenia across cultures.* California: University of California Press. 127–138.

Sousa, A.J. (2016). Diagnostic neutrality in psychiatric treatment in North India. In Luhrmann, T.M. and Marrow, J. (eds.). *Our most troubling madness: Case studies in schizophrenia across cultures.* California: University of California Press: 42–55.

Spandler, H. and Poursanidou, K. (2019). Who is included in the Mad studies project? *Journal of Ethics in Mental Health.* Open Volumer: 1–20.

Spivak, G.C. (1988). Can the subaltern speak? In Nelson, C. and Grossberg, L. (eds.). *Marxism and the interpretation of culture.* Urbana: University of Illinois Press: 271–313.

Spivak, G.C. (2010). Subaltern Studies: Deconstructing historiography. In Guha, R. (ed.). *Subaltern studies IV: Writings on South Asian history and society.* New Delhi: Oxford University Press: 330–363.

Srivastava, K., Chaudhury, S., Bhat, P.S. and Mujawar, S. (2018). Media and mental health. *Indian Psychiatry Journal.* Jan–Jun; Vol. 27, No. 1: 1–5.

Stewart, E. and Roy, A.D. (2014). Subjectification. In Teo, T. (ed.). *Encyclopedia of Critical Psychology.* New York Heidelberg Dordrecht London: Springer: 1876–1880.

Stiedenroth, K.S. (2014). Female, young, unmarried: The role of positionality while conducting fieldwork in Pakistan. *Orient Anthropology.* Vol. 14, No. 1: 81–95.

Sugiman, T., Gergen, K.J., Wagner, W. and Yamada, Y. (2008). The social turn in the science of human action. In Sugiman, T., Gergen, K.J., Wagner, W. and Yamada, Y. (eds.). *Meaning in action: Constructions, narratives and representations.* Japan: Springer. 1–20.

Summerfield, D. (2012). Afterword: Against "global mental health". *Transcultural Psychiatry.* Vol. 49, No. 3: 1–12.

Summerfield, D. (2013). "Global mental health" is an oxymoron and medical imperialism. *British Medical Journal.* Vol. 346: f3509.

Sweeney, A. (2016). Why Mad Studies needs survivor research and survivor research needs Mad studies. *Intersectionalities: A Global Journal of Social Work Analysis, Research, Polity, and Practice.* Vol. 5, No. 3: 36–61.

Sweet, P.L. and Decoteau, C.L. (2017). Contesting normal: The DSM-5 and psychiatric subjectivation. *BioSocieties.* Vol. 13, No. 1: 103–122.

Szasz, T. (2007). *The medicalization of everyday life: Selected essays.* New York: Syracuse University Press.

Szasz, T.S. (1974/2010). *The myth of mental illness: Foundations of a theory of personal conduct*. Harper Perennial: New York, London, Toronto, Sydney, New Delhi, Auckland.

Szmukler, G. (2019). "Capacity", "best interests", "will and preferences" and the UN Convention on the Rights of Persons with Disabilities. *World Psychiatry*. Feb; Vol. 18, No. 1: 34–41. DOI: 10.1002/wps.20584. PMID: 30600630; PMCID: PMC6313688.

Thara, R. and Rajkumar, S. (1993). Nature and course of disability in schizophrenia. *Indian Journal Psychiatry*. Vol. 35: 33–35.

Thirthalli, J., Venkatesh, B.K., Kishorekumar, K.V., Arunachala, U., Venkatasubramanian, G., Subbakrishna, D.K. and Gangadhar, B.N. (2008). Prospective comparison of course of disability in antipsychotic-treated and untreated schizophrenia patients. *Acta Psychiatrica Scandinavica*, 1–9. DOI: 10.1111/j.1600-0447.2008.01299.x

Thirthalli, J., Zhou, L., Kumar, K., Gao, J., Vaid, H., Liu, H., Hankey, A., Wang, G., Gangadhar, B.N., Nie, J.-B.N. and Nichter, M. (2016). Traditional, complementary, and alternative medicine approaches to mental health care and psychological wellbeing in India and China. *Lancet Psychiatry*. DOI: 10.1016/S2215-0366(16)30025-6.

Thompson, S.A. (2002). My research friend? My friend the researcher? My friend, my researcher? Mis/informed consent and people with developmental difficulties. In van den Hoonaard, W.C. (ed.). *Walking the tightrope: Ethical issues for qualitative researchers*. Toronto, Buffalo, London: University of Toronto Press: 95–106.

van Dijk, T.A. (2001). Critical discourse analysis. In Schiffrin, D., Tannen, D. and Hamilton, H.E. (eds.). *The handbook of discourse analysis*. USA and UK: Blackwell Publishers Ltd.: 352–371.

van Dijk, T.A. (2007). Ideology and discourse: A multidisciplinary introduction. Available at: http://www.discourses.org/UnpublishedArticles/Ideology%20and%20discourse.pdf.

van Dijk, T.A. (2015). Critical discourse analysis. In Tannen, D., Hamilton, H.E. and Schiffrin, D. (eds.). *The handbook of discourse analysis*. Second Edition. UK: Wiley Blackwell: 466–485.

van Os, J., Kapur S. Schizophrenia. Lancet. (2009) Aug 22; 374(9690): 635–45. DOI: 10.1016/S0140-6736(09)60995-8. PMID: 19700006.

van Os, J. and Tamminga, C.A. (2010). Introduction. In Tamminga, C.A., Sirovatka, P.J., Regier, D.A., van Os, J. (eds.). *Deconstructing psychosis: Refining the research agenda for DSM-V*. Arlington, Virginia: American Psychiatric Association.

Voronka, J. (2015). Troubling inclusion: The politics of peer work and "people with lived experience" in mental health interventions. Unpublished doctoral dissertation. Toronto: Ontario Institute for Studies in Education.

Voronka, J. (2016). The politics of "people with lived experience"- experiential authority and the risks of strategic essentialism. *Philosophy, Psychiatry, & Psychology*. Vol. 23, No. 3/4: 189–201.

W.H.O. (2012). Risks to mental health: An overview of vulnerabilities and risk factors. Available at: https://www.who.int/mental_health/mhgap/risks_to_mental_health_EN_27_08_12.pdf.

Walia, S. (2021). Pegasus, a blemish on democracy. *The Hindu*, Monday, August 2:7. Available at: https://www.thehindu.com/opinion/op-ed/pegasus-a-blemish-on-democracy/article35670524.ece.

Wallcraft, J. (2009). Recovery – a double-edged sword? Presented at the Critical Psychiatry Network Conference, Norwich, UK, 21 June 2009 (http://www.mentalhealth.freeuk.com/Doubleedged.htm.) Downloaded on 22 Aug, 2018.

Whitaker, R. (2015). *Anatomy of an epidemic: Magic bullets, psychiatric drugs, and the astonishing rise of mental illness in America*. New York: Broadway Books.

Wispelwey, B. (2021). Decolonizing public health requires an epistemic reformation. *Health and Human Rights Journal*. Vol. 23, No. 1: 297–299.

Woods, A., Hart, A. and Spandler, H. (2019). The recovery narrative: Politics and possibilities of a genre. *Culture, Medicine and Psychiatry*. DOI: 10.1007/s11013-019-09623-y.

World Health Organization (2000). World Health Report. Available at: https://www.who.int/whr/2000/en/whr00_en.pdf.

Yarris, K.E. and Ponting, C. (2019). Moral matters: Schizophrenia and masculinity in Mexico. *ETHOS*. Vol. 47, No. 1: 35–53. DOI: 10.1111/etho.12226

INDEX

Note: **Bold** page numbers refer to tables; *italic* page numbers refer to figures and page numbers followed by "n" denote endnotes.

AD *see* Advance Directive
Addlakha, R. 53, 54
Advance Directive (AD) 165–169, *168, 170*
agency 18, 19, 28, 30, 80, 96, 101, 104, 105, 117, 122, 123, 131, 132, 135, 137–139, 140, 147, 150, 151, 157, 181, 182; **183, 185, 189**; epistemic 184, 189
agenda, setting 16–17
Ahearn, L.M. 139
Arbour, L. 145, 148
Arstein-Kerslake, A. 152
Asylums (Goffman) 45n8
atomistic approach 18
Australia 39
autobiographical power, gaining 132–133, 182
autonomy 94, 140
awareness about "mental illness," creating 172–173

Barrett, A.E. 108
barriers to recovery 27, *168*, 180–183
Bayetti, C. 40, 53
Beresford, P. 10
Bindhulakshmi, P. 53, 54, 92
bipolar disorder 4, 5, 14, 19, 20, 200
Borg, M. 39, 56, 136
bounded beings 111–117
Boyle, M. 81
Brahmakumaris 90n9
Burke, K. 83
Burr, V. 47
Burstow, B. 14, 135

CAM *see* complementary and alternative medicines
Campbell, L.A. 165–166
"Can the Subaltern Speak?" (Spivak) 42
Carel, H. 43, 44, 97, 132
Casanova, G. 30
Cassell, E.J. 180
CCRH *see* Central Council for Research in Homoeopathy
CDA *see* Critical Discourse Analysis
Central Council for Research in Homoeopathy (CCRH) 203
Central Mental Health Authority (CMHA) 155; constituting 173–175
Chalia, D.S. 201
Chamberlin, J. 42
clinical recovery 38, 148, 183
CMHA *see* Central Mental Health Authority
coloniality 30–33, 55, 168, 184–186
complementary and alternative medicines (CAM) 100, 101
Conrad, P. 186
continuity, maintaining 137–139
Convention of Rights for Persons with Disability (CRPD) 27, 28, 58, 146–150, 157, 166, 172–178, 182, 184; Article 1 149n4; Article 3(a) 149n5; Article 3(b) 149n5; Article 4 149, 149n6; Article 4(1)(b) 149n7; Article 4(1)(g) 149n8; Article 5 150; Article 5(2) 150n9; Article 8(1)(b) 150n10; Article 9 150; Article 9(2)(c) 150n11; Article 9(2)(f) 150n11; Article 12 150–152; Article 14 152, 152n21;

Article 19 153; Article 19(b) 153n22; Article 19(c) 153n22; Article 21 153, 153n23; Article 23 153; Article 23(b) 153n24; Article 24 153, 153n25; Article 24(c) 153n25; Article 24(d) 153n25; Article 26(2)(b) 153n26; Article 27(1)(a) 153n27; further provisions facilitating recovery in 152–154
Cooke, M. 77
Correll, C.U. 200
Costa, L. 5
course-corrections 119–120
Critical Discourse Analysis (CDA) 26, 66–70, 180
critical pedagogy 58
Critical Psychiatry Network Conference 37
critical theory 50, 190
CRPD see Convention of Rights for Persons with Disability
curiosity 4, 9, 51, 57, 59, 100, 131

D'Arcy, M. 96
Darwin, K. 74
Das, V. 53
Davar, B.V. 16n15
Davar, B.V. and Lohokare, M. 188
Davidson, L. 35, 38
De Bhailís, C. 152
decolonial 187, 190
decoloniality 8, 55, 179–191
decolonizing 179, 187, 189, 191
Descartian mind-body dualism 163
Deshpande, S.N. 53
design 8, 27, 56, 58–61, 157, 176n76, 190, 204
Dhanda, A. xv, xvi, xvii, 10, 111, 130, 149, 157, 162, 177n78
Diagnostic and Statistical Manual of the American Psychiatric Association (DSM) 18, 164
diagnostic labels 1, 7, 14–16, 18, 46, 52, 58, 76, 81, 137
diagnostic reductionism 14
diffusion 16, 71
disability 6, 9–13, 16, 21, 22, 27, 32, 52, 53, 58, 59, 64, 146, 148–163, 181, 197–200; definition of 21; psychiatric, nature of 21; psychiatric "treatment" and 160–161
disability studies (DS) 10–13, 16, 58

discourse, and recovery 133–135
discourse analysis 26, 75, 146
"disease management" approach 155, 157
distress: children's, parental response to 91–96; as diagnosis, reconfiguring 83–96; as illness 5; as illness, misrecognition of 183–184; as mental illness 17–19; as psychosis, misrecognition of 4
distributive epistemic injustice 150n12, 163
Dotson, K. 57, 137
Dressler, W.W. 139
drug-free recovery paradigm 37, 182
DS see disability studies
DSM see Diagnostic and Statistical Manual of the American Psychiatric Association
Duncombe, J. 65

emancipatory 4, 5, 7–9, 11n12, 12, 13, 16, 21, 26, 32, 33, 36, 49, 54, 183, 184, 187, 190
emancipatory research paradigm 1, 11, 17, 25, 58, 59, 60, 63–64
emancipatory-survivor research 58
empowerment 41, 64, 65, 177
epistemic agency 189
epistemic ignorance 62, 185
epistemic injustice 2, 26, 31, 43, 44, 97, 132, 150n12, 163
epistemic marginality 98
epistemic privilege 17, 31, 43, 56n1, 87
epistemic reformation 187, 191
epistemic viability 56
epistemic violence 42–45, 57, 185, 188
epistemology 6, 18, 33, 57, 178, 187, 190, 191
experience 1, 4, 5, 6, 10, 14, 20, 21, 22, 24–26, 29–34, 36–38, 42–47, 50, 51, 53–57, 59, 64–66, 79, 81, 84, 85, 103, 116, 117, 121, 122, 128, 131, 134, 136, 137, 156n35, 174, 191; coloniality 30–33; definition of 29; illness 30–33

Fairclough, N. 3, 25, 68–70
family's assistance towards recovery 140
Faulkner, A. 65
Feuchtersleben, E. von 23
Fields, M.J. 109

Fish, S. 49
Flynn, E. 152
Foucault, M. 29n1, 30, 45, 51, 68, 75, 77, 81, 186, 189
framing futures 188–191
Frank, A. 46–47
Fraser, N. 188
freedom 86, 104, 113, 115, 127, 149n4–6, 167, 168, 181, 189, 190; of choice 171; political 167, 168, 190; of the slave 167
Freire, P. 71
Freud, S. 74
Fricker, M. 26, 43, 44, 150n12, 163, 167–168

Gadamer, H.-G. 49
gain 1, 64, 139, 142, 189
Gammeltoft, T.M. 102, 103
Ganim, J.M. 74–75
Geddes, A. 65
gender equality 111
gender inequality 111
Gergen, K.J. 14, 18, 47–50, 52, 111, 141
Global Mental Health Action Plan 2013–2020 177, 177n81
Global Mental Health Movement (GMHM) 130, 155, 164, 190
Global North 34n2, 39, 40, 189
Global South 189
GMHM see Global Mental Health Movement
Goffman, E. 80, 124; Asylums 45n8
Gooding, P. 159
governmentality 45–46
Greenberg, J.S. 93

Hacking, I. 50, 52
Hahnemann, S. 201–203; Organon, The 201–202
Hardt, M. 68
Harper, D. 37, 39–40, 81
Hay, C. 57
Helman, D.S. 41
help seeking 55, 61, 74, 78–83, 119, 165
hermeneutical injustice 43
holistic approach 18
homeopathic mental health establishment 201–205
Hyden, L.- C. 57

identity power 43, 132
identity prejudice 43, 44, 46, 58, 97, 102, 185
Illich, I. 186
India: Department of Social Welfare 170; human sciences "mental health" research in 52–55; Mental Health Act of 1987 40; Mental Healthcare Bill of 2013 40; Ministry of Health and Family Welfare (MoHFW) 155n31; New Pathways, New Hope 40, 175; recovery in 40–41; "Recovery Model" 40–41; 67th Annual conference of Indian Psychiatric Society 40
Indian Mental Healthcare Act 2017 (MHCA) 27, 147, 148, 154, 155, 157–160, 162, 175–178, 181, 182; Advance Directive (AD) 165–169, 168; awareness about "mental illness," creating 172–173; Central Mental Health Authority, constituting 173–175; nominated representative 169–171; psychiatric "patient" at par with another 171–172; and recovery 163–175
Ingleby, D. 87, 122
Ingram, R. 12
injustice 6, 8, 13, 181: epistemic 2, 26, 31, 43, 44, 56n1, 97, 132, 150n12, 150; hermeneutical 43; testimonial 43, 44, 184
"insider-outsider" space 5, 58, 59
internal colonialism 30

Jadhav, S. 53
Jain, S. 175, 176, 177n77
Janks, H. 69, 70
Japan 39
Jara, R.S. 31
Jarman, J. 117
Jessop, J. 65
Jones, N. 131n1

Kane, J.M. 200
Kaur, H. 201
Kidd, I.J. 43, 44, 97, 132
Kiossev, A. 31
Kisely, S.R. 165–166
knowledge, as social construction 50–51, 76, 189
Kopelowicz, A. 38, 41
Kuhn, T. 49

Lachman, M. 36, 37
language 6, 13–15, 17, 25, 26, 31, 47, 49, 50, 51, 63, 66–68, 74, 76, 84, 86, 159, 176, 185; madness, representation of 14–15
Larsen-Barr, M. 136
law 8, 12, 25–28, 34, 55, 58, 72, 79, 145–178, 181, 184, 186–188
LeFrancois, B.A.: *Mad Matters* 12
legal capacity 148, 150, 151, 152, 152n19, 158, 165, 169, 172, 175, 176, 182
legal-policy barriers 181
Liberman, R.P. 38, 41
Liegghio, M. 42–43
Linguistic Philosophy 67
Link, B.G. 124
Locke, J. 187
Luhrmann, T.M. 53, 109–110

MacGregor, H. 116
macro-environment 58, 79, 127, 146–148, 167
mad 7–9, 10n11, 12, 13, 25, 28, 189
Mad Matters (LeFrancois, B.A., Menzies, R. and Reaume, G.) 12
madness, representation of 10, 12, 14–15
Mad Studies 5, 7, 10–13, 54, 73n1
Major, C.H. 6
Manchanda, R.K. 201
manic depression 5, 19
marginality 2; epistemic 98
marginalization 10, 15, 43, 55, 175
marital families 101, 102, 108–111
Marrow, J. 53, 110
Marx, K. 74
Mathias, K. 111, 116
Maulik, P.K. 172–173
medical pluralism 28, 148, 150, 157–159, 163, 167, 171, 203
medical plurality 157, 163, 171; legitimizing 158–159
medical regimen, stabilizing 96–101
Medina, J. 97
mental health 3–8, 10, 11, 13, 16, 17, 19, 20, 22, 24–29, 32–38, 40, 41, 45, 52, 56, 59, 71, 72, 79, 91, 96, 116, 125, 129–133, 143, 147, 153, 156, 160, 162–166, 169–178, 188; micro-politics of 180–181; praxis 6–7; representation 6–7; research 6–7

mental health policy (MHP) 147, 148, 175–178
Mental Health Review Boards 155
mental illness 4, 5, 7, 10–12, 17, 20, 21, 26, 42, 79, 92, 93, 99, 112; awareness about, creating 172–173; and capacity to make decisions 164–165; diagnosis 23, 77; distress as 17–19; experience of 29–30; knowledge about "treatment" 161–163; medical plurality, legitimizing 158–158; permanent 155–163; reality 25; recovery 35–40, 42; representation 25; rights-based approach 159–160; as socially constructed discourse 51–52; transient 155–163; treatment orientation in 130
mental incapacity 166
MHCA *see* Indian Mental Healthcare Act 2017 (MHCA)
MHP *see* mental health policy
micro-environment 146, 147–148, 181
micro-politics of mental health 148, 178, 180–181
Mignolo, W. 189, 190
Mills, C. 155
Minotaur 179, 180
Morrison, L.J. 189–190
Morrow, M. 40
Myers, N.A.L. 132

Nandy, A. 31
narrative 1, 5, 14, 16, 20, 21, 23, 25, 26, 28, 34, 43, 46–48, 51, 56–61, 64, 66, 69, 72, 75, 77, 81, 87, 94, 99, 106, 126; analysis of 66–70; inquiry studies 57–58; progressive 141; reconstructions 140–142; regressive 141–142; stability 141; surrender 46–47; through a lens of subjectivation 77–83
National Homoeopathy Research Institute in Mental Health (NHRIMH) 203; mental health research 204–205
National Institute of Mental Health Recovery, England 38
Negri, T. 68
neuroleptics 19, 197–200
NHRIMH *see* National Homoeopathy Research Institute in Mental Health

nominated representative (NR) 165, 166n53, 169–171
NR *see* nominated representative
Nunley, M. 53, 91

O'Donnell, A. 32
Oliver, M. 63–64
ontology 14, 18, 20, 35n3, 52, 53–54, 153, 155, 157, 174, 178, 182, 188, 189
Oosterhoff, P. 102, 103
oppression 3, 8, 10, 13, 16, 21, 31–33, 115, 191; intersectional 33; systemic 31
Organon,The (Hahnemann) 201–202
Ortner, S.B. 139

Padmavati, R. 53
parental response to children's distress 91–96, 103–105
Parker, I. 19, 84
Parsons, T. 22n19, 47
paternalism 129, 157
Pathare, SZ. 102
pathology 35, 68, 74, 75, 76, 78, 88, 89, 99, 107, 128, 138
patienthood 3, 9–11, 16, 20, 29, 33, 38, 41, 42, 54, 55, 78, 82, 96, 128, 129, 132, 133, 135, 136, 141, 146, 160, 174, 182, 185, 199
patient–psychiatrist, relationship between 30, 31, 44, 76, 78, 80, 96, 97
Pattadath, B. 32
peer(s) 4–8, 15, 26, 54, 56–70, 73, 75, 77, 83, 124, 127; challenges of meeting 64–65; demographic profiles of 193, **194**; encountering 23; families 59–60; knowledge 56–59, 62; meeting 59–60; relationship with 65–66; research 15
personal context 19–20
personal recovery 5, 20, 38, 48, 132, 133, 183
persons with disabilities (PwD) 10, 27, 146, 148–152, 153n22, 153n25, 181
Phelan, J.C. 123, 124
Pilgrim, D. 24, 36, 39
Pinto, S. 53
Pisani, A.M.O. 31
polanco, m. 190n4
political freedom 167, 168, 190
Political power 187

Pompili, M. 102
Porter, M. 31
positionality 5–13, 58
poststructuralist theories 74
Poursanidou, K. 10
power dynamics 66, 81
praxis 6–7
prejudice 6, 43, 44, 46, 57, 58, 97, 102, 114, 123, 149, 150n10, 164, 172, 173, 185, 190; identity 43
progressive narrative 141, 142
propaganda 16, 98, 174, 185, 191, 203n3
propagation 16
psychiatric dependence, existing 136–137, 182
psychiatric diagnosis 4, 8, 9, 10, 21–22, 24, 31, 50, 67, 68, 76, 77, 77n5, 79, 81, 95, 98, 101, 104, 128, 182, 204
psychiatric disability, nature of 10, 21–22
psychiatric gaze 131–133, 144, 145, 181, 185
psychiatric morbidity 15, 130
psychiatric "patient" at par with another 171–172
psychiatric subject 11, 34, 73–126, 128, *195*
psychiatric "treatment" and disability 160–161
psychiatrist–" patient" relationship 30, 31, 44, 76, 78, 80, 96, 97
psychiatry, recovery movement in 38–39
psycho-centrism 161
psychopathology 37n4
psychosis 1, 37, 50, 58, 59, 64, 66, 71, 124, 127, 128, 137, 160, *196*; definition of 23–24; descent into 83–96; diagnosis of 35, 71; distress as, misrecognition of 4; recovery from 3–28
psy-knowledge 89, 191
psy-professionals 6, 15, 39, 81, 89, 130, 132, 149, 151n18, 153, 155–157, 173, 180, 181, 183, 189, 190
psy-professionals recovery 130
psy-professions 12, 45, 184, 191
Puras, D. 159
Putnam, R. 116
PwD *see* persons with disabilities

qualitative research 19, 26, 27, 60

Ranganathan, S. 53
realities 3–28, 35, 38, 44, 45, 49,
    51–53, 74, 76, 77, 81, 96, 99, 101,
    110, 117, 123, 128, 134, 137;
    constructed nature of 47–48; mental
    illness 25; social 26
Rebughini, P. 77
reciprocity 64, 116, 137
recognition, decolonizing 179–191;
    barriers to recovery 180–183;
    instituting recovery 182–183; reasons
    for 183–188; representation 184–186
recovery 27, 56–58; clinical 38;
    comprehension about, gaining 20–21;
    definitional issues 163–164; definition
    of 23–24; discourse and 133–135;
    divergences on 36–38; exiting
    psychiatric dependence 136–137;
    factors contributing to 135–142;
    as goal 129–133; in Indian context
    40–41; instituting 182–183; maps
    of 71–72; as medical outcome 35;
    method of 39–40; MHCA and 163–
    175; movement in psychiatry 38–39;
    personal 38; personal aspects of 41;
    politics of 34–42; psy-professionals
    130; as reclamation project 35;
    relational aspects of 111–117
recovery-focused approach 157
"recovery from" 3, 4, 18, 20, 28, 35,
    36, 40, 134, 135, 183, 196
"recovery in" 36, 196
Recovery Narrative 131, 132, 140,
    142, 182
regressive narrative 141–142
rehabilitation 21, 23, 36–38, 40,
    77, 132, 135, 143, 147, 150, 153,
    155n31, 173, 178, 181, 183;
    "best" treatment as fighters of
    "schizophrenia," search for 120–123;
    continuity amidst transitions 118–
    119; course-corrections 119–120;
    outcomes of 117–123
relational aspects of recovery 101–117;
    bounded beings 111–117; marital
    families 108–111; parental response
    103–105; siblings, participation of
    105–108
relational aspects of research 61–66
representations 3–28, 7, 31–34, 44, 49,
    50, 53, 54, 57, 68, 75, 81, 128, 135,
    156, 173, 174, 177, 184–186; mental

illness as 25; self-representation 7–9,
    25; social 16
resilience 39, 107, 131
resistance 11, 13, 33, 39, 80, 83, 91,
    133, 138, 187, 188–191
responsibility 19, 35, 108, 114, 118,
    137–140, 142, 144, 161, 170, 188,
    205
Reynolds, F. 89
right to information (RTI) 162
Roberts, G. 81
Roe, D. 36–38
Rorty, R.M. 67
RTI see right to information
Rubio, J.M. 200
Russo, J. 10

Sarin, A. 169, 175, 176, 177n77
Savin-Baden, M. 6
schema 63, 68, 78, 96, 124, 129
Scheper-Hughes, N. 110
schizophrenia 4, 14, 21, 22, 36, 51, 53,
    61, 70, 107, 110, 112, 119–123, 126,
    142, 200, 204, 205, 205n9; "best"
    treatment as fighters of, search for
    120–123
Schneider, J. 186
Scott, J.W. 29, 32
Scott, S. 65
self-colonizing 31
self-determination 39, 129–132
selfhood 74, 114, 123, 133
self-reification 122
self-representation 7–9, 11, 25, 68,
    135, 174
Sholl, J. 186
siblings, participation of 88, 92, 93,
    102–108, 110, 111, 120, 123,
    139, 212
Slade, M. 118
SLE see systemic lupus erythematosus
Smith, D. 45
social capital 116, 125, 143, 200
social construction 18–20, 26, 45, 47,
    52, 58, 63, 66, 67, 189; emergence of
    48–50; knowledge as 50–51
social constructionism 49, 52, 67
social constructionist theory 48
social defeat 132
social inequality 40, 82
social psychiatry 36
social psychology 16, 48

social reality 8, 21, 26, 81
social representations 6, 16, 53, 57, 68
sociolinguistics 76
Sood, A. 53
Sousa, A.J. 53, 111
Spandler, H. 10
Speed, E. 37, 39–40
Spivak, G. 57; "Can the Subaltern
    Speak?" 42
stability narrative 141
State Mental Health Authorities 155,
    156n35, 173, 174
stigma 6, 19, 53, 59, 93, 96, 102, 132,
    142–144, 147n3, 164, 172, 173, 181;
    as barrier 180; response to 123–126
structuralist theories 74
subaltern 31, 185
subject 19, 74–77, 80, 128–129
subjecthood 45–46, 55, 77, 127, 128,
    183
subjectivation 45–46, 74–79, 127, 183;
    narrative through a lens of 77–83
survivor 4–9, 11, 13, 15, 17, 34, 37, 38,
    42, 54, 58, 65, 122, 146; research 6
Sweeney, A. 5–6
systemic lupus erythematosus (SLE)
    198, 199
systemic oppression 31
Szasz, T. 39, 186

Tamminga, C.A. 24
testimonial credibility 184
testimonial injustice 43, 44, 184

Thompson, S.A. 65–66
Tian, X. P. 199
treatment 3, 9, 11, 15–17, 22, 29,
    30, 35–38, 197–200; alternatives,
    searching for 99–101; gap 40, 130;
    knowledge about 161–163

UK/Britain 39, 133
UN-CRPD 26–28, 58, 146, 146n2,
    147–163, 166, 171, 173, 174–177,
    181, 182, 184
US 38, 39, 103, 106, 109, 131, 133, 136

van Djik, T. 68, 69
van Os, J. 24
Voronka, J. 32, 174

Wallcraft, J. 37
Weisser, J. 40
W.H.O. see World Health
    Organization
will and preference 144, 147, 151, 152,
    157, 159, 165, 167, 172, 176, 182
Woods, A. 132
World Health Organization (W.H.O.)
    111, 158, 177

X, Tisha 190n4

Zea, L. 189
Zhang, X. 199
Ziv, T. 132
Zola, I. 186

Taylor & Francis Group
an **informa** business

Taylor & Francis eBooks

www.taylorfrancis.com

A single destination for eBooks from Taylor & Francis
with increased functionality and an improved user
experience to meet the needs of our customers.

90,000+ eBooks of award-winning academic content in
Humanities, Social Science, Science, Technology, Engineering,
and Medical written by a global network of editors and authors.

TAYLOR & FRANCIS EBOOKS OFFERS:

A streamlined
experience for
our library
customers

A single point
of discovery
for all of our
eBook content

Improved
search and
discovery of
content at both
book and
chapter level

REQUEST A FREE TRIAL
support@taylorfrancis.com

Routledge
Taylor & Francis Group

CRC Press
Taylor & Francis Group

For Product Safety Concerns and Information please contact our EU
representative GPSR@taylorandfrancis.com
Taylor & Francis Verlag GmbH, Kaufingerstraße 24, 80331 München, Germany

www.ingramcontent.com/pod-product-compliance
Lightning Source LLC
Chambersburg PA
CBHW060250220326
41598CB00027B/4052